Total Transformation of the Body, Mind & Spirit

Total Transformation of the Body, Mind & Spirit
Discover How to Achieve Complete Healing, Transformation and Balance in All Areas of Your Life

Mariana Chiarella & Pablo Ricciardi

All Rights Reserved. No portion of this book may be reproduced, stored in a retrieval system, or transmitted in any form or by any means-electronic, mechanical, photocopy, recording, scanning, or other-except for brief quotations in critical reviews or articles without the prior permission of the author.

Published by Game Changer Publishing

ISBN PAPERBACK: 978-1-963793-33-8
ISBN HARDCOVER: 978-1-963793-34-5
ISBN DIGITAL: 978-1-961189-88-1

DEDICATION

To our beloved Sergito,
wherever you are living your next adventure.

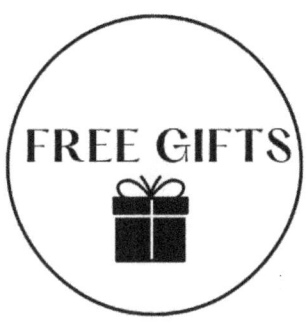

DOWNLOAD YOUR FREE GIFTS

Read This First

Just to say thanks for buying and reading our book, we would like to give you a few free bonus gifts, no strings attached! Scan this QR Code or visit **https://www.marianandpablo.com/free-gift-download** to access your free gifts.

Total Transformation of the Body, Mind & Spirit

Discover How to Achieve Complete Healing, Transformation and Balance in All Areas of Your Life

Mariana Chiarella & Pablo Ricciardi

Acknowledgments

We want to express our heartfelt Gratitude to our all-time teachers/ heroes/ mentors.

- **SERGIO MEDINA** (our dear friend and REIKI Master - God Bless his memory and soul to keep teaching us from a higher plane).

- **Dr. DEEPAK CHOPRA** - Whose books paved the road to our own self-discovery and learning. - **Dr. BRUCE LIPTON** - Who wrote such incredible books to understand that we create our own experiences in life through our perception.

- **Dr. JOE DISPENZA** - Who discovered the powerful force of our thoughts that can bless us into total transformation or doom us into total physical and emotional limitations.

- **Dr. GREGG BRADEN** - An amazing scientist in constant search for our true meaning and power in this world.

- **MORRNAH NALAMAKU SIMEONA and Dr. HEW LEN** - Great exponents and teachers of Ho'oponopono.

- **LOUISE HAY** - Whose unconditional love taught us to be kinder to ourselves (may God continue to guide her higher than the stars!).

- **WAYNE DYER** - Without whom, we wouldn't have learned to appreciate each part of ourselves).

- **MARIO CORONA** - Whose guidance helped us put together this book.

- **CRIS CAWLEY** - Whose patience, hard work and kindness breathed life into our dream of sharing all our experience with you.

Disclaimer

This book contains the opinions and ideas of its authors. It is intended to provide helpful and informative material on the subjects addressed in the publication. It is sold with the understanding that the author and publisher are not engaged in rendering medical, health, or any other kind of advice or professional services in the book. The reader should consult his or her own competent medical or health professional before drawing inferences from anything listed in this book and its contents. This book also is not intended to serve as the basis for any decisions or health recommendations. The authors and publisher specifically disclaim all responsibility for any liability, loss, risk, personal or otherwise, that is incurred as a consequence, directly or indirectly, from the use and application of any of the contents of this book.

Preface

Congratulations! We are super happy to share this path of transformation with you. If you have the courage and the will to apply what you will find here, you can achieve the following:

HOW TO HEAL YOUR BODY

- Learn simple ways to increase your energy.
- Know the ancient art of healing that is Ayurveda.
- Discover the 5 forces of the Universe that dominate everything that exists.
- How to improve your metabolism naturally to rejuvenate your entire body.
- How to recognize your psychophysical biotype (DOSHA) in order to implement specific balance plans for you.
- You will learn simple breathing exercises that are very beneficial for your health.
- How physical activity directly affects your overall health.
- Amazing benefits of drinking hot water.
- And how a simple age-old habit can make a world of difference in your life!

HOW TO HEAL YOUR MIND

- Learn to deal with and tame your inner demons.
- How to achieve cardiac coherence in less than five minutes.

- Learn to be responsible and get rid of the blame.
- How to identify your ingrained limiting beliefs in order to modify them.
- How to learn to forgive through the HUNA and Ho'oponopono philosophy.
- How to get in touch with your inner child in order to heal it.
- How to find your true "Why" in life through a simple exercise.

HOW TO HEAL YOUR SPIRIT

- Know the true way to bless: the hidden art to release tensions and pains of the soul.
- You will learn simple and effective techniques to meditate (we give you guided meditations).
- Discover your *True Self*.
- You will learn to manifest what you want (Sankalpa - Ancient powerful technique of visualization and manifestation).
- How to connect with your intuition.
- How to align your body, mind and spirit.
  … and much more!

Success Stories

Here are a few success stories from some of our clients across the globe.

"Both Mariana and Pablo are two people who dedicate their lives to study and the search for tools that serve as support for people. With a lot of passion for what they do, full awareness and commitment to the other. Healing from the soul is possible and necessary. They are for me, a guide for difficult moments."
- **Cecilia Calafell**

"Mariana and Pablo are excellent coaches. Their ability to teach is surprising, clear, simple, and very professional. They have managed to penetrate the souls of those who listen to them with each word and make special changes in each one. What perhaps very few know is that they are incredible people and great friends, whom you will never forget." - **Silvia Federici**

"At a very difficult time in my life. I had an apprenticeship that helped me to overcome many obstacles. Breathing exercises and guided meditations accompany me every day of my life. Thank you, dear teachers, Mariana Pablo. I currently use it with each patient" - **Ingrid Nadir**

"For more than ten years, Mariana and Pablo, with a deep and delicate vocation, commitment and joy, have built a path for the greater good. They're already in legacy mode... from their lives to ours. They are constant researchers. With their knowledge to connect with our creation. They help me a lot to solve situations that allow us to transform and aim to have that long-awaited "better *every day"* in ourselves, to share it and grow, expanding consciousness with the ancient Ayurveda through food, meditation, and above all truthfulness of course. always experimenting and supervised with its transparency. With the desire to grow together in this new world. Many congratulations on the launch of your book Total Transformation." - **Arminda Moscoso**

"I want to dedicate these words of gratitude to my dear teachers who have lit the lanterns of love for myself. My journey accompanied by Pablo and Mariana was an awakening to gratitude, kindness and love. My transit of spiritual awakening was so wonderful at the hands of these wonderful people. The prism of life today is different, although I have taken the steps, accompanied by so much love in his teachings, they have left a huge mark on my life and on my heart. Because after I changed, everything changed. My family and I love you very much! I bless the existence of my dear teachers. - **Elena Meza**

I met Mariana and Pablo in 2016. They are excellent teachers, very professional, but also affectionate and cordial. I have learned a lot from you. I love you so much. Thank you! - **Antonia Morel**

I met Mariana and Pablo when I participated in an Ayurveda course and really from the beginning I understood what I had been looking for a long time: the right people to understand what I was doing. They were and still are amazing teachers. With them, explanations were never lacking as many times as necessary. I appreciate everything they taught me that I have applied it and continue to apply it in my daily routine today. - **Estela Tita**

I met them in 2015 and it was a great find. Mariana and Pablo are excellent in transmitting the fundamentals of Ayurveda, Ayurvedic massage and REIKI. They are generous with all the information. They disclose easily. I thank life for being able to cross paths with them. Thank you, Mariana and Pablo. Namasté
- **Francisco Miliarese**

With Mariana and Pablo I got to know Ayurveda, the Science of Happy Life and I discovered the secrets of well-being. I learned ethics, equanimity, values, positivity to solve difficulties, knowing that we are not alone on this planet and developing from our interior to the exterior to modify behaviors rooted in the past with good results in the present towards the future with teaching in a framework of love and I respect all living beings. - **Jorge Pazos**

"I have enjoyed the program very much. Mariana and Pablo are great coaches. Excellent material and resources; concise and accurate information contained in the course, thank you!" - - **Pilar Yanez**

"Magnific! I've been wanting to learn these ancient arts for a long time and the program is wonderful." - **Kevin Alejandro Torres Rodriguez**

"Mariana is engaging and has a wonderful warmth and clarity. The subject matter speaks deeply to the place that I am in my life, practically and spiritually and I strongly feel that this is the right path to enable me to further my healing and spiritual journey." - **Sarah-Jane Franklin**

"I really liked the program! It's super interesting. In addition, Mariana and Pablo convey tranquility, peace and harmony." - **Ana Bailles Isart**

"This program helped me refresh and put into practice the necessary steps to be centered and calm!!!" - **Lina Yanet Ferrer Taboada**

"Excellent program!" - **Hector Luna**

"I have long wanted to learn more about Ayurveda. Thank God I found this course. I know myself better according to the Doshas and what they imply. I appreciate this opportunity that Mariana and Pablo have created to improve my quality of life." - **Viviana Rolon**

"Everything I have learned in this program is incredible. I thank coaches Mariana and Pablo for being able to make this a reality." - **Tania de la Cruz**

"This program is a beautiful symphony of tradition, culture and universal principles." - **Dimitri Snowden**

"There is a before and after in my life after finishing this program." - **Sandra Guerra Aguirre**

"Fantastic! The most intensive and profound Ayurveda program I have ever seen." - **Vanessa De Jesus**

"The experience with this program was truly enriching. It allowed me to acquire much more knowledge than I had imagined and I have already put it into practice. I feel incredible! Thank you, thank you, thank you." - **Paola Montarzino**

"Thank you for the really positive messages in this course! They are truly wonderful to listen to!" - **Emma Frank**

"Mariana and Pablo's program is very complete, very pleasant when studying it, super well explained. I am delighted with the coaches. Thanks!" - **Luján Meram**

"Incredible explanation, brilliant. This program is the best way I have ever come across to understand human growth. Thank you!" - **Maria Ines Cuadra**

"This is very informative and the most in-depth program I've done on Ho'oponopono. I've taken Joe Vitale's course. I definitely preferred this one. What I like most is that you can tell these instructors genuinely care about people and want the best for everyone. Mariana and Pablo truly go out of their way to give life changing information. Again, great program, and ALOHA!" - **Tasha Danvers**

"Excellent program. Clear, direct and to the point. The meditations are beautiful and you feel the vibration change immediately!" - **María Belén Benavente**

"This program is life changing and I highly recommend it to everyone!" - **Courtney Grace**

"Everything I ever wanted to know about Ho'oponopono." - **Rian Pelati**

"I loved the dynamic and the loving and simple way in which Pablo and Mariana explained each of the concepts. They helped me get to know myself and understand how to return to balance. I have already started slowly to make changes in my life. Thanks for sharing your knowledge!" - **Pat Luna**

"This program came exactly when I needed it most. It just feels perfect! Highly recommend it!" - **Nardus Grobler**

"I loved the voice and presence of the coaches. Infinite thanks for your love and availability." - **Silvia Montalvo Colorado**

"Truly LOVED this program!" - **Hala Ashrf**

"This program is fantastic! It is so detailed and Mariana has a beautiful voice that really touches my soul. Every time I listen to her speak, my inner child is nurtured." - **Argyro Maria Veniou**

"I loved the program. It has given me a lot. I have taken note of everything that resonated with me to apply it in my day to day life. Thank you Mariana and Pablo. They are great!" - **Maria Lado**

"I loved the program. The instructors are very nice; I love their good humor. The information is complete and very interesting. I will continue to apply what I have learned in my day to day life. Thank you so much for everything." - **Lorena Delgado González**

"I really liked this program. The most important thing is to know the reason why we study something. What led me to choose this program is that I was seeking emotional peace. During the course I began to use what I have learned in my life. In the moments when I felt like getting angry, I remembered what I had learned and it made me lower the intensity of my emotion, transferring it to the area of my responsibility and then I gradually found the stability I was looking for. Highly recommended!" - **Sergio Guerrero**

"It came at the very right moment and is fantastic!" - **Natalia Willey**

"What an amazing program… Thank you so much for bringing us to the light!" - **Dilani S.**

"Mariana and Pablo have a lot of energy and help keep the program moving forward. Each of the lessons was perfect, just as it had to be for my moment. Thank you very much!" - **Andrea Valín Fontão**

"Such a beautiful program! Enjoyed every minute of it." - **Susan MacKay**

"This is a fabulous program! I have loved what I have learned. They explain it very clearly. I am so glad I signed up!" - **Karla Ochoa**

"I'm a massage therapist currently working through the grief of losing a loved one to suicide. I found this course to be very helpful in future interactions with clients and helping me move on from that tremendous loss. Thank you so much for this new found tool. Appreciating all the time and effort that went into this." - **Emily M.**

"Mariana and Pablo, Thank you so much for such a fantastic program. I think I fell in love with Mariana's voice :) It was soothing and made me look forward to each lesson. I hope to practice the techniques daily and bring in some changes in my life. I love the way the program was conducted; it was simple, easy to *follow and made with a lot of love and affection. Thank you for this incredible opportunity to learn one of the key truths in life. Lots of love."* - **Piyali Ghosh**

"Loved the explanations. I'm working on personal growth and forgiveness. When I first read about ho'oponopono I couldn't find a lot on the subject. As soon as I started working on myself. There you were!!!! I bought the Zero Limits and stopped more than half way through. I was so confused. Yours was way better. Highly recommend it!!!!! -**Bobbie Reihe**

"This program exceeded my expectations. Excellent!" - **Lidia V.**

"I loved the program! I am beginning to apply what I have learned and I am beginning to feel the changes. Thank you!" - **Fred Urrutia**

"Mariana and Pablo are great teachers! This program is dynamic, profound and very useful." - **Pablo Kaswalder**

"It seems to me a program that is most necessary in the life of each person. Many times we do not remember that we have to nurture our soul as we nurture our body and unload it from garbage and remains that both we and our ancestors have left us. With much love and without guilt. Thank you, thank you, thank you, thank you, for sharing this knowledge, Mariana and Pablo!" - **Dolores Hernández**

"Lots of useful information. I would highly recommend this program to anyone interested in learning about having a better life! The instructors are great and as practitioners they include important hands on information making the learning process easier and more approachable. Very happy to have invested in this program." - **Dayamí Velázquez**

"Mariana and Pablo are very prepared people and have the knowledge to be able to convey it." - **Jose Jimenez**

"I have been fascinated by this program. I do not regret at all trusting Pablo and Mariana. I thank you very much for this valuable information and this teaching. It has allowed me to know myself better and to know what is good for me and how to have a balanced and healthy life. Very happy!" - **Zaira Salazar Castro**

"I really enjoyed Mariana and Pablo's program. I will definitely be continuing with the practice :) Thank you Mariana and Pablo! I love You both." - **Andrea Horn**

"This program is great, very deep and profound! I really like it!" - **Victoria Schnare**

"I love this program and the affection that Mariana and Pablo transmit in each class. You can see the effort and dedication in every detail. I will put into practice everything I am learning and thus improve my life. Congratulations for your work and positive energy ☺." - **Belén Valencia**

"I loved this program. All the contents are well explained and with a lot of love." - **Fatima Rojas**

"It was an amazing program! I learned so much and enjoyed every minute of it. Highly recommended." - **Orli Degani**

"I love this! I am learning a lot. Thank you very much Pablo and Mariana for your dedication and love. Super geniuses!!!" - **Irene Chi**

"It is a wonderful program. The teachers explain each of the lessons very well and everything is very clear. I recommend it 100%." - **Ramiro Monge**

Table of Contents

Acknowledgments .... *ix*
Disclaimer .... *xi*
Preface .... *xiii*
Success Stories .... *xv*

Introduction - The Best, Always 1

Part 1: Body 5
   Chapter 1- Temple Of The Soul 7
   Chapter 2 - Ayurveda & The 5 Forces of The Universe 19
   Chapter 3 - Restore Your Energy 31

Part 2: Mind 41
   Chapter 4 - The Power of Your Thoughts 43
   Chapter 5 - Take Responsibility - Create Healthy Emotions 53
   Chapter 6 - Ho´Oponopono - The Ancient Art of Healing 63

Part 3: Spirit 79
   Chapter 7 - Huna Principles To Change Your Life 81
   Chapter 8 - The Power of Forgiveness 95
   Chapter 9 - Manifest What You Wish 103

Conclusion - A Death and a Birth 123

Introduction

"Health is a state of complete harmony of the body, mind and spirit. When one is free from physical disabilities and mental distractions, the gates of the soul open..."
- **B. K. S. Iyengar**

It does not matter if you are healthy, sick, alone or in a relationship; if you meditate or not or if you have ever tried to change your life, this book will help you and it will give you the road map to your true self and healing. This is an inner path of self-discovery and understanding so that every day, word by word, you begin to understand a little more about yourself and how to connect with that space of peace, wisdom and healing that dwells within you.

We are Mariana and Pablo, coaches in health and natural healing through different disciplines of life. We have studied the ancient art of life, which is **Ayurveda**, a natural way of connecting with the body and health; **Ho'oponopono**, a profound healing technique through forgiveness and inner discovery; **Reiki, Meditation**, among others.

For the past twelve years, we have been teaching courses, programs, workshops and seminars focused on health and inner healing. We are co-authors of the Best Seller *Tu También Puedes Sanar (You can heal too)*, and creators of *Algo Alternativo (Something Alternative)* and *Medicina Ayurvédica (Ayurvedic Medicine)*, two programs dedicated to alternative and complementary ways to lead a healthy and balanced life.

WHY?

Why did we write this book? Why did we write **Total Transformation of the Body, Mind & Spirit?**

In a world where everything is partial, everything is fast, immediate, where most of the solutions are incomplete, we need a total solution, a total transformation, body, mind and spirit. We all need a tool, a blueprint, a framework, a roadmap to transform our lives not only in a fragmented way, but in a complete way because we are not isolated people, nor are we pieces joined together—we are a whole.

All our body systems and all the parts of our life are united in a holistic and complete way. Our whole being functions in an organized and synchronous way to perfection. By dividing it, we become ill because we are in imbalance and disharmony. The phrase *"divide et impera,"* (divide and conquer) exemplifies what we want to share with you.

With this book, we do not want to divide anything, but to unite all the parts of your being. By unifying all our parts, we achieve true healing, in a total and profound way.

The only true conquest is the conquest of our fears, doubts, anxieties and weaknesses. Bringing love, understanding and awareness to every corner of us, in order to recognize them and integrate them into what we are: complete, unique and perfect beings.

In this book you will see that most of the time, the words are written in the first person plural, "we."

Why is that? Because we have written it together. Many of the experiences you will learn about here have been lived together, but you will also notice that at some points you will find that there are words written in the first person singular. This is because we are going to tell you stories or experiences that we have lived individually. When the story merits, you will find spaces dedicated exclusively to Pablo's stories and Mariana's stories, where we will share with you our own real experiences, those of our family and students, which will help you to better understand the content we've developed.

We will also give you practical exercises so that you can begin to apply them in your daily life because knowledge, if it is not applied, is not useful at all, it does not transform, and our promise with this book and with everything we are going to share here is to transform your life.

No matter what you've been told or believe, **you deserve the best life** in the universe.

You deserve the best, always.

Since we were kids, we have heard a phrase that, today, we have reinvented: when you greeted a neighbor with an affectionate "*Have a nice day!*" The answer was always the same. "*God willing.*" This phrase always struck us.

Why would God *not* want you to have a good day? Why would the universe want you to suffer or get sick?

Both God and the universe, or the creative force (whatever you want to call it), wants you to be happy and live with all the abundance and prosperity you deserve. And in this way, achieve your mission in life for which you have been created and brought into this world.

So, when you find yourself in situations of stress, crisis and even illness, ask yourself this question: What *does life want to teach me? How can I transcend this in order to be happy?*

Let's say it again. **You deserve the best life in the universe, you deserve to be happy in every moment of your life.**

If you are one of those people, like us, who are in search of something more: better relationships, whether family, personal and work; a better perception of your financial situation and abundance both material and spiritual; having higher energy levels, feeling healthier and going to the doctor less; having a healthy and sound body and managing to connect with your spiritual world, achieving a communion with your true self, your intuition and creative force... Then this book is for you!

If you want to transform your life, this book was written for you.

The three parts of this book will help you connect you with your totality, with your body, with your mind and emotions and also with your spiritual world. Each chapter of this book will guide you to achieve what you want to transform in your life. This information will help you connect with a space of wisdom, so you can discover that you are whole, complete and perfect. You just need the knowledge to do this.

We will guide you to discover the keys that open the doors to your personal transformation.

Here is a great idea. We recommend you have **a notebook or a notepad** to help complete the exercises we will propose throughout these pages in a deep and conscious way.

In each chapter, we will address universal knowledge for the deep and total healing of your body, mind and spirit, and we will share stories that will help you better understand the practical way to apply all the information we share with you.

We welcome you to your *Total Transformation.*

Part 1: Body

Chapter 1

*"Dissolve your whole body into Vision:
become seeing, seeing, seeing"*
- Rumi

Today you begin a new life. We want you to know that this book was written with love and with the desire for you to be prosperous, healthy and happy. So get ready to take the quantum leap you were looking for to achieve everything you set out to do.

To achieve change in our lives, we must first know *where* we are.

Knowing your starting point allows you to better prepare for the change you want to achieve. **And all change first begins within**, then it manifests itself outside. So we start with a question, *What do you want to transform?*

While you are thinking about the answer to this question, we are going to introduce you to one of the great secrets that opens the door to self-discovery—**Ayurveda**.

Our body is the temple of the soul. What does this mean? It means that we are complete beings and that every part of our being is equally important. Many times the soul, or the emotions, or the thoughts, or our memory, or our intellectual part is taken as more important, and we leave our body aside.

That's why we started with the phrase, "The temple of the soul."

Our body is a temple and deserves to be respected. It deserves to be cared for and it deserves to be treated with all the love you can give. Our body has certain characteristics and each of us is made the same, but in different proportions. That is why each one of us is unique and irreplicable.

The Body is the Temple of the Soul.

How much importance do you give to your body today? How much time do you dedicate during the day or during the week to take care of your body? And what do you think taking care of your body really means? Many people think that taking care of the body is to focus on exercise, rest or solely on nutrition. In reality, the body is a compendium of many daily habits. Eating is one of the most important.

For Ayurveda, the oldest existing medicine, which was born in India more than five thousand years ago, **"Food is everything that enters through the senses."** In other words, our body is nourished by what it hears, what it sees, smells, touches and tastes

All the experiences that surround us are part of our daily nourishment.

This means that we are constantly feeding on the things we see, the things we experience and the company of the people with whom we share our daily lives, not just the food we put in our mouths.

Our body takes everything as food in order to survive and also to nourish itself with experiences, to evolve and to maintain itself in a state of constant transformation.

"Food is everything that enters through the senses."
- **Ayurvedic proverb**

This Ayurvedic proverb totally changes the perspective we had about food, don't you think? Starting from this principle, we must consider how we eat. You may have a fairly healthy and balanced diet, but *where* do you usually eat? Is it bright, quiet and peaceful? What do you usually do while eating? Do you see or hear anything? Do you have company?

For Ayurveda, each of us is a whole. We are not separated parts. And we perceive reality through our five senses which we cannot shut off. We absorb everything we perceive and feel from the outside world. Each thing we absorb becomes part of us, affecting us in a good or a bad way (bringing balance or imbalance to our health and daily life)

So mindful eating involves not only having a greater understanding of the food we eat, but taking notice of everything around us as we eat, the things we hear, the things we see, the things that surround us, the time of year and the time of day.

So now we ask, *What is your diet like?*

Some time ago, one of our students, Norberto (47), made a comment to us about food. During one of our seminars, he told us, "I understand that it is healthier to eat well, but when I get together with friends, we eat a whole pork and drink wine and whiskey and I feel great, I don't have any stomach discomfort or heartburn. But when I eat with my wife a little salad or something healthy, I feel bloated and upset. What is going on there?"

"What's going on with your wife?" We asked.

Everyone laughed. But after the funny moment, we explained what we are going to share with you now... This is one of the greatest secrets of Ayurveda—**Everything is food.** Therefore, one of the maxims of Ayurvedic nutrition is not to eat when we are angry or sad, much less cook in these states, because **our vibration impacts and affects everything that is near.**

A great Ayurvedic axiom says, *"It is preferable to eat the wrong food with the right attitude rather than the right food with the wrong attitude."*

Our food is everything we think and feel. That is why, for Ayurveda, food is a ritual of nutrition where we take new energy and let go of that which is stagnant or no longer serves us.

It is preferable to eat the wrong food with the right attitude, then to eat the right food with the wrong attitude.

In this book, we are not going to go too deep into Ayurveda because it would take us several volumes, but we do want to give you a small synthesis of everything we have been applying and teaching in our programs.

The depth of this medicine is that it treats the person, the patient, as a whole: body, mind and spirit. And in the case of the body, we must nourish it, bless it, and give it the best food. We must give it the best care so that it can develop in fullness and in its totality.

This medicine considers the following: **health is not the absence of disease**, but a state of fulfillment and happiness, where one can develop all of one's gifts, talents and qualities to their fullest expression.

And we can extend this definition a little more. Being healthy also involves the balance of our energies, digestion, metabolism and proper evacuations, the effective functioning of our sensory functions, a radiant psyche, healthful emotions and a satisfied self.

Health is a state of fulfillment and happiness.

An ancient axiom says, *"Ayurveda was born so that human beings can discover their inner reality."* That is, the connection we have with our own health, in a state of fullness, is the key way in which we will be able to discover who we truly are.

By bringing to light our fullest potential, we can live in bliss, being who we were meant to be in this life, accompanied by a healthy body, a balanced mind and a fulfilled spirit.

Ayurveda allows us to know who we really are, how our energies act in our body and how we can find a balance and a natural equilibrium that keeps us in a state of happiness. It also allows us to understand that imbalances are part of life and that they are learning experiences through which we discover who we are. Why? **To be able to self-manage our health,** to be able to connect in a natural way with what our body, mind and spirit need.

Ayurveda was born so that human beings can discover our inner reality.

We are going to share with you a personal story as an example so that you can understand how easy it is to find balance once you have the right knowledge.

Mariana's Story

I was finishing college when I met Ayurveda and realized that my life was full of imbalances.

In addition to the study hours, I had three jobs teaching English in kindergarten, elementary school and in company courses

I was under deep stress, but I did not realize it. I had a hard time digesting my food. I had very little sleep and it was never a complete rest. I also had a hard time focusing on college. I suffered from horrible migraines almost every week and took painkillers to try to reduce them, but to no avail.

But the thing that was affecting me the most was family conflicts. I had a hard time having a good relationship with my family and my partner because I was incredibly exhausted, and I did not understand why.

Why did I feel so bad if I was doing all the things I loved? I loved my job, I loved being with my students, I loved being in college.

But, despite all the love I put into every single thing I was doing, it was not enough to be able to combat my daily stress and anguish.

It took me a long time to realize that all my discomfort was nothing more than the stress of overexertion. It took me almost three years to turn stress into strength. But I finally succeeded.

No one wants to change. When we are doing something we love and we encounter obstacles, we tend to think, "Okay, I can handle this." And when the obstacles pile up, when negative stress begins to cover every corner of our life, we keep thinking, "No problem. I think I can handle it."

This is incredibly WRONG.

We cannot handle it all. And it is healthier to accept that we can no longer suffer than to continue to endure a situation that hurts us and hurts us. Why? Because what the outside world thinks of us weighs more heavily on us than taking charge of the pain of our inner world.

It was hard for me to understand that I had to make changes in my life, but luckily the changes following the principles of Ayurveda were very simple. They were small things that I adapted from my daily routine and today I keep repeating and respecting them. My life changed dramatically. I was able to start sleeping better, I started to enjoy my food more, I started to adjust my daily schedule to be able to enjoy my family's company more.

I started to feel in a better mood at work, to have a better relationship with my coworkers and everything came naturally.

Maybe, like Mariana, this has happened to you. You may have reached such a point of stress that you feel that your whole life is out of order. Or maybe it is happening to you right now. What is important and what we want to share with you is that there is an easy and simple but, at the same time, very profound solution to give your body the balance and health it needs.

It is essential to connect with self-knowledge because, through self-knowledge, one discovers what we truly need. In Mariana's case, she realized that with a lot of movement energy, adding more movement (traveling a lot to and from her different jobs) was throwing her off balance.

A Vedic principle says, *"Things alike increase their energy, and opposite qualities bring balance."* Through this knowledge, we will realize what we need to bring balance to our life. And this is reflected in an integral health; health of the body as well as of the mind and spirit.

The body is the first door, the first barrier that is usually affected by any external stress. Therefore, in the case of Mariana, a very creative person, very cerebral, with a predominance of the energy of thought, speech and communication, which in Ayurveda is translated as Air and Movement energy, moving a lot was affecting her in a very negative way.

Later we will explain what the different energies of Ayurveda consist of, but it is key that you understand that it is actually very simple to return to balance. We simply need to be able to understand how our energies work, how you work, and how your body works.

We often get used to suffering and this is what we do not want for you. We do not want you to get used to suffering or constant stress. Life is much more than that. And above all, this temple that is your body deserves that you fully enjoy every single thing you do because every experience is a new opportunity to learn, to learn who you are. It is important to remember that we came to this life to enjoy it, not to suffer from it.

In Ayurveda, everything happens naturally. According to this medicine, life is a gradual, tolerant and loving process. In the same way we should be with ourselves and especially with our own body.

We often get angry because we discover that our body is failing because we feel pain, when in fact, we do not realize that the body gives messages. It warns us when something is not working properly. And yet, instead of listening to it, we commonly cover up those messages and wait for something to break or hurt so that we can go to the doctor or focus on our health.

You have a perfect body here and now. At this moment, how much attention and respect are you giving to this temple that belongs to you?

Ayurveda allows us to focus in a loving way on our health, not only when health fails, not only when there is an imbalance, but every day of our lives.

In Mariana's case, she learned to love herself and her body and to give it what it needed. But first, by understanding how it works, what it was needing and what its "Achilles heels" were, its imbalance indicators.

It is vital to be able to know ourselves in order to understand what things we should incorporate into our daily routine that bring health.

We will now share with you a very simple but very beneficial exercise. It is a **pranayama**. A pranayama (*prana*: energy / *ayama*: control) is an exercise that allows us to regain control of our vital energy through breathing. This exercise consists of achieving square breathing. It is called square because it will be done four times.

You can do this breathing exercise even if you have never practiced a pranayama exercise before. There are countless pranayamas, but this is one of the most simple and accessible to start implementing now.

WHAT DO YOU GAIN BY DOING THIS EXERCISE?

This pranayama allows you to calm and regulate the autonomic nervous system (ANS), which regulates involuntary bodily functions such as temperature, heart rate, widening of blood vessels, among other things.

This simple exercise can help you reduce blood pressure, generating an almost immediate feeling of calm. In addition, by slowly holding your breath, you can cause carbon dioxide (CO_2) to accumulate in the blood. An increase of CO_2 in the blood improves the cardioinhibitory response of the vagus nerve when you exhale and stimulates your parasympathetic system. This produces a feeling of calm and relaxation in your mind and body.

And, as if all this was not enough, it also helps you reduce stress and improve your mood. It is ideal for imbalances such as generalized anxiety disorder, panic attacks, post-traumatic stress disorder (PTSD), and depression. If you suffer from insomnia, we also recommend you do this exercise since by calming the nervous system before going to sleep, you achieve the proper relaxation for a good rest.

EXERCISE 1

Inhale through your nose in four times (counting to four), hold the air for four seconds, exhale, and hold the air again for four seconds. Repeat this process as many times as you want.

You can do this type of breathing at any time of the day, and you can do it even when you are at work. Simply take a few minutes to relax.

This breathing allows us to bring our attention back to our breathing and become aware of the air coming in and out and the way our body expands to take in air and contracts when we let it out.

"The soul lives in the breath."
- Buddha

Breathing is the key to bring us back to the present moment, but also to control our emotions. When you have a moment of stress, anger, irritation or frustration, use this square breathing exercise to bring you back to the present, to bring you back to the coherence of this present moment and to ground you in this moment of awareness and growth.

BREATHING EXERCISE

https://www.marianandpablo.com/square-breathing

We are going to share with you another simple exercise. This exercise is very interesting and very special because it is recommended by Dr. Bruce Lipton, an expert in Cell Biology.

Dr. Lipton has conducted studies and written a great book called, *The Biology of Belief*, where he explains how our beliefs and thoughts affect our body. According to Lipton, everything you believe in has generated and manifested the body you have today.

This exercise is simple and very effective in bringing coherence and balance to both body hemispheres.

HARMONY EXERCISE

Sit comfortably and, if possible, barefoot. Cross one ankle over the other and then cross your arms. Keep your arms crossed with your ankles crossed and simply breathe deeply in this posture.

This way, by crossing our arms, what we do is to bring all our attention to our cerebral hemispheres unification. This will allow you to restore coherence and mental balance.

Many times we think or react using more the capacity of one brain hemisphere than the other.

With this exercise, we are able to restore our balance to give us a greater coherence and a greater connection with our being in a total and not fragmented or divided way.

You can do this exercise several times during the day here: https://www.marianandpablo.com/cerebral-hemispheres-balance

Chapter 2

"The human body is the chariot; the Self, the person who drives it; thought is the reins, and feelings are the horses."
- Plato

We would like to begin this chapter with a true story.

Pablo's story

The gloomy Dr. V.

When I was about twenty-one years old, I had to do my annual check-up. Taking advantage of the fact that there was a doctor known by my family a block away from my house, I took the results to him. As soon as I entered, I was greeted by a tall, hairless person with a rather dark voice who said, "Welcome," in a cold and very protocol-like manner. He reviewed the studies and added, "The studies are fine. Keep them for when everything is wrong." He continued reviewing, and after a few moments, he "gave me" a phrase that remained ingrained forever in my mind, "You should know that life is a long and hard race towards death."

When I heard those cold, sad and almost perverse words, I was stunned. I greeted him, dismissed him and said, "This cannot be life. Life has to be something else." And thanks to this dire prognosis I started looking for something alternative and that is where I discovered the wonderful medicine that is Ayurveda.

Your life is not a race towards death. Your life is not a road to pain, suffering and eventually death. Your life is much more than that. That does not even need to make up a major part of your life, because your life is so much more than you can imagine.

And why did we start with this story? Because thanks to Pablo's terrible experience, he was able to learn about Ayurveda. But in your case, you do not need to go through a traumatic event to take advantage of all the benefits of this wonderful medicine.

Here are some of the Ayurveda pillars for you to apply in your life.

The five forces of the universe

This Ayurvedic theory is called "the five elements of nature" and is a fundamental pillar from which the following theories and principles are then created, and which relate to the creation of the universe.

The material universe is created through five elemental forces, or five elements, ranging from the subtlest to the densest. This means that everything that exists in the material universe, everything that you can see and touch in your life, is created thanks to the conjunction of these five forces: **ether, air, fire, water and earth.**

Everything we can see and touch is composed of these five forces. There are just some that have more proportion than others. For example, a tree has a higher proportion of earth energy and water than of ether or air. But all things that exist will always be created through these five elements. This theory gives us the guideline that we are all created with the same ingredients.

What differentiates us from one another is the proportion in which these elements are conjugated. In other words, we are all made of the same material, but our essence is unique and unrepeatable.

There is a phrase we want to give you, "**You are the compendium of the universe.**" It can be related to a phrase of Rumi that indicates, "**You are not a drop in the ocean; you are the ocean in a drop.**"

This phrase is coupled with this Ayurveda principle because many times we think that the universe is something external, that nature is something outside of us and in reality, each one of us is an inherent part of nature. We are a part that cannot be separated from nature. Because just as the trees, the plants, the animals are created through these five elemental forces, so is your body. We are nature. We are the Universe.

You are not a drop in the ocean, you are the ocean in a drop

And taking up Pablo's story, as sad as this medical encounter was, it shows us that we are often wrong in the way we perceive ourselves. We believe that we are something broken and damaged, something that does not work quite right and something that needs to be repaired. In fact, from Ayurveda, we are all part of nature, and nature is perfect as it is.

Nature is dynamic. It is not something stagnant, but a continuous movement of learning vibrating in constant health and wellness. And despite the moments of imbalance, Nature and Life always find their natural balance again.

In nature, we can observe the four seasons of the year. We observe that the summer passes from the heat to the humidity and cold of autumn to reach the winter cold and winter turns into spring for a new summer to begin.

Consequently, nature goes through these seasons and these seasons bring with them an effect on nature. There will be animals that are more prone to a hot climate and others to a cold climate. There are foods that the earth grows in times of cold and in times of warmth. And in the same way, your body does not react the same during the heat as it does during the winter. For this reason, we should not consume the same foods in winter as in summer.

Every season, every moment of our life, brings with it a special learning. So we return to the phrase, *"You are the compendium of the universe."* The whole universe is within you because within you are the same ingredients with which the stars are created, with which the trees, lakes, rivers, mountains and animals are created.

Everything that is part of nature contains these same ingredients. Therefore, we return to this particularity that belongs to you, that you are unique and unrepeatable. Why? Because each element within you is going to behave in a different way. You have a special proportion of these five elements. In Ayurveda, this is called **"Dosha."** Dosha means "natural constitution." We also call it natural psychophysical constitution because it refers to the way these energies manifest in your body, in your mind and in your whole being.

When we become aware of how these energies behave within us, we can make a self-evaluation and a plan to bring balance with respect and love. With understanding, we learn how to create healthier routines that will adapt perfectly to our special needs. And we also understand better our general difficulties in life.

Why are some foods better for us than others? Why are there times of the day when we feel more creative or more productive? And why are there times of the day we find more tiring? Do you find it hard to get up early or to stay up late?

It is very interesting to be able to know ourselves in a profound way because self-knowledge is the key to transformation, starting with acceptance and deep understanding. When you manage to understand who you are, you have the key to change your whole world and to understand the learning moments that will have the greatest impact on your life.

When you understand who you are, you have the key to change your whole world.

A wrong view of life is to think that we are all the same and that we all think and act in the same way. This is inaccurate because each one of us manifests these natural energies, these five elements of nature, in different ways.

Some people tend to relate more to thinking and others to feeling. Are they weird to do so? Are they missing something? Are they incomplete? No, definitely not.

Each of us manages to manifest our energy in a unique and special way. In this way, each one of us has things to learn, but most of all we have things to accept about ourselves. When we manage to understand what our primordial nature is and which energies are more predominant, it is much easier to find the key to achieving a healthy and harmonious life.

In the previous chapter, we shared with you Mariana's story, who, despite loving her job, realized that stress was generating her great physical and mental imbalances.

What was the key to transforming that stress? How could it be that, despite doing what she loved, she was having such a hard time?

When Mariana managed to understand her true nature, her *Dosha,* she noticed that she possessed the influence of the elements ether and air energy. This translates into making Mariana a person filled with constant mental activity—lots of thinking, movement and creativity but also fear, doubt and anxiety. An Ayurvedic maxim states that akin energies alike bring imbalance, but opposite energies bring balance. Mariana understood that all the movement in her life (having three different jobs and traveling all the time from one workplace to the other) had generated a profound imbalance in her daily life that did not allow her to sleep, digest, or even think properly.

That's the magic of Ayurveda—discovering who we really are.

In this regard, Pablo realized the importance of discovering his own value, of finding that life is much more than pain or suffering. That life is something that we are actually discovering day by day and that our being is complete and perfect, in a constant state of learning to bring complete harmony.

Every moment of imbalance, for example, when we get sick, is simply a *learning experience so that the body can naturally return to its natural balance.*

This learning moment shows us that everything in life is dynamic and that just as things move, they return to their course.

In the same way that winter appears in nature, then spring comes, followed by summer and autumn, to return to winter, there are stages through which we must go through in life. They are experiences that need to be lived. This principle of Ayurveda -the five forces of the universe- allows us to understand that **everything changes and that this change is part of life**.

We will briefly describe each of the characteristics of these elementary forces of nature. It is important to remember that these five forces are part of all creation. The Rishis (ancient enlightened men in Vedic philosophy) discovered that **everything that exists in the material universe, the physical world, is composed of these five energies. And these five energies are also within you.**

ETHER / AKASHA

Space, or *Akasha,* is the place that allows all energy and all matter to manifest. For something to happen, first, there is a space that is prepared for it to happen. For example, in the female body, for a baby to gestate and grow, the female body prepares itself for the arrival of a new life each month, creating blood and tissue to cover the lining of the uterus to hold the fertilized egg or zygote. This ether energy is fundamental for all matter to manifest. And it is the first force, the subtlest, that will allow the next energy to develop.

AIR / VAYU

The energy of air, or "Vayu" in Sanskrit, is an energy of movement. Once we have a space ready for creation to manifest, there is a movement that will generate the beginning of creation, and this movement is given and represented by the air element.

This air within our body is reflected in the thoughts and movement of our whole body. Thus, the lung's expansion and contraction, blood movement, etc., is the manifestation of the Vayu, air energy. Everything that moves in our body contains the primordial energy of this elemental force.

FIRE / AGNI

Space brings about movement and movement generates a friction of energy. This friction creates warmth and heat, and this heat is reflected in the element of fire (*Agni* in Sanskrit). This energy of fire within our bodies can be found in the constant transformation that takes place in the metabolism process through the separation of food into nutrients and waste. Everything we see, everything we ingest, is transformed within us. And for this transformation to take place, the energy of **Agni** is vital because it allows us to discriminate between what is useful from what is not necessary. Our body constantly makes this natural discrimination. According to Ayurveda, we should perceive life in this same way—separating the experiences that serve us from those that harm us.

WATER / APAS

Water is the energy that allows union and consolidation to take place in our whole body. Water allows the communion of all energies. It also creates a density that will result in the possibility of experiencing the sensations of our body. Emotions and feelings are related to this water energy. Water, then, provides us with nutrients that will keep our body together in constant union and perfect balance, where emotions can flow in a natural way.

EARTH / PRITHVI

The densest elemental energy is the energy of the Earth. Earth represents solid matter and the structure of the universe and it gives form to the human body and to all of creation. The structure provided by the earth element is the conduit through which all the other elements flow. In the human body, this energy translates into our entire bone structure, muscles and tendons.

Now, let's consider this. Are any of these energies unnecessary or unimportant? Could you imagine your body without structure, without transformation, or without movement? Could you have a body if there was no space to receive it or no form to create it?

Each of these forces then makes it possible to create and give life to the body we have today. Naturally, each of us has a special body, a perfect body that will have characteristics completely different from another person. These five elemental forces are coincident with the five senses, that is, just as these forces of the elements allow the creation, they also allow us to connect with the material and physical world through our five senses in the following way.

Space allows us to develop the sense of *hearing* in Sanskrit **"Shabdarth."** Water allows us to relate to the sense of *taste*, also called **"Rasa,"** the taste for life. Air allows us to relate to *touch*, to realize that this physical and natural world can be touched. We can appreciate it through the skin. In Sanskrit, it is called **"Sparśa"** and refers to the connection of our body with material life. Earth allows us to connect with the sense of *smell*, **"Gandha,"** in Sanskrit, which allows us to discover that material life has particular smells and aromas.

Fire or "Agni" connects us with **"Rupa,"** the sense of sight. Sight allows us to transform everything we see into personal appreciation. Everything you see in the material world has a special perception because it is seen through your eyes, through the lens with which you give life a specific meaning.

Thus, each of these five elements (connected to the five senses) allows us to transform our lives and we can become aware of the fact that life is a living experience, an experience that is lived, heard, tasted, touched, smelled and seen. And our body, being also a physical and material experience, has these five elements that allow its creation and its perfect functioning.

This book's purpose is to help you transform your life and to help you realize the true value of your life.

In this first part, we talked about your body. In this chapter, we addressed the importance and value of your body, unlike all others, because you are unique and unrepeatable and because your body is formed with a special percentage of the five forces that create the universe; of these five elements through which all creation is generated. **Everything that exists in the universe also exists within you.**

Now, it's time you get to know who you really are. We propose you discover the special proportion of these five elements through a **"Dosha"** questionnaire. This is a very simple Ayurvedic questionnaire to discover your true energy and the exact predominance of the elements in you. Through this knowledge, you will be able to understand which element is in greater and lesser proportion and how these energies work.

Knowing this will help you understand what things you will need to bring balance to your life, to be able to find a natural harmony, far from suffering, far from illness and far from pain.

We need to understand that life has been created for us. And that our body is also a dynamic experience that deserves respect and self-knowledge. So with this test, we propose you get to know yourself a little better and discover what elements predominate in your body.

*"Life's not happening **to** you. Life's happening **for** you."*
- **Tony Robbins**

We hope you can connect with this test in an honest and sincere way. It is very important that you take this test several times. You can even do this questionnaire with someone close to you (a partner or a member of your family), someone who knows you. The answers need to be as objective as possible in order to get the most accurate result possible. There are no wrong answers.

Remember, you are the compendium of the universe.

https://www.marianandpablo.com/ayurvedic-test

Take charge of your life and achieve optimal health with our Ayurveda Program. Ready to transform your life? Enroll now!

https://www.marianandpablo.com/ayurveda-program

Appearance	VATA	PITTA	KAPHA
Complexion	skinny, irregular	medium, proportioned	well-built, bulky
Weight	easy to lose and difficult to gain	easy to lose and easy to gain	difficult losing, easy to gain

Skin	dry, rough, cold, opaque, dull	soft, oily, warm, faired, reddish	thick, oily, cold, pale, white
Sweat	very little, even when it is hot	abundant, especially when it is hot	moderate, constant
Hair	dry, curly, dark	thin, straight, fair (tendency to recede or bald)	shiny, oily, abundant, brown or dark
Teeth	big, crooked, protruding	medium, yellow	strong, white
Eyes	small, dry, dull	blue, piercing	big, attractive, with thick lashes
Appetite	variable, irregular, very little	strong, intense	steady
Preferred Flavour	sweet, sour, salty	sweet, bitter, astringent	spicy, bitter, astringent
Thirst	variable	strong, excessive	very little
Evacuation / elimination	dry, hard, constipated	regular, tends to diarrhea	slow, oily, thick
Weather	prefers hot	prefers cold	prefers season changes
Physical activities	very active	moderate	lethargic, passive
Vigor	little, tends to overexert	medium; tends to use a lot when competing	a lot; uses very little energy

Sexual drive	variable	usually intense	little
Thought process	mostly verbal	logic and sensory related; visual thinking	emotional related
Mind process	restless, very active	smart, discerning, sharp, acute	calm, slow, smooth
Negative Emotion	fear, insecurity	anger, jealousy	greed, attachment
Positive Emotion	enthusiasm	joy, passion	compassion, temperance
Faith	variable	strong, fanatic	stable, durable
Memory	learns and forgets easily	learns fast and forgets slowly	learns and forgets slowly
Dreams	scary, about flights, jumping or running	fire related; angry, violent, of war	romantic and water related; rivers, sea, lakes
Sleep habit	irregular, usually interrupted; tends to suffer from insomnia	little but efficient	heavy, long
Speech	fast, talkative, loquacious, rambling	sharp, direct, precise, straightforward	slow, cautious, boring, monotonous
TOTAL:			

Chapter 3

"Mastering the power of your mind can be more effective than the drugs you have been programmed to believe you need."
- Bruce Lipton

Do you know what the key to life is? In this chapter, we are going to talk about the key to life and how we can transform our life following very simple steps.

Do you know where life comes from? Where is the capacity with which we can measure our life? It is the **energy**. Energy is the basis and source of life.

So where does energy come from? Have you ever thought about it? The answer is simpler than you think. Energy comes from your *cells*. According to Cell Biologist *Bruce Lipton*, Ph.D., the human being is not a body, not a single life entity, but a community of more than fifty trillion cells.

Each of us, each human being, is a community of cells perfectly organized in the various systems that make life function optimally. It is the cells that promote our health and provide us with the energy we need to live from day to day. And there are three fundamental and vital factors that cells need in order to remain stable, healthy and productive: **oxygen, hydration and elimination.**

Oxygen

All cells require oxygen in order to live. Without oxygen, cells die. It may sound simplistic, but the reality is much simpler than we imagine, although no less important.

In 2019, three great specialists were awarded the Nobel Prize in Medicine for their contribution to the relationship of cells and oxygen: William G. Kaelin, Sir Peter J. Ratcliffe, and Gregg L. Semenza. The laureates state that oxygen sensing is fundamental to a large number of diseases. The discoveries made are of fundamental importance to physiology and have paved the way for promising new strategies to combat anemia, cancer and many other diseases. This information deserves to be recognized and deserves our attention.

We all breathe, but are we really aware of the importance of good breathing for our biological functions? Have you ever thought that good oxygenation would help you strengthen your body against cancer? Well, if you did not know before, you do now. **The first sin we commit is ignorance. The second is foolishness**. That is, today you have invaluable information that you did not have before and, because you did not know, you could not apply it. But today, we give you the power to start generating health in each of your cells, bringing your consciousness to your breathing.

The first sin we commit is ignorance.
The second is foolishness.

Before we continue, we would like to do a practical exercise with you. Place the soles of your feet flat on the floor. Try to keep your back straight and your spine as aligned as possible. Relax your shoulders and neck and breathe. Breathe slowly and deeply. Try to fill your body completely with air until you feel the air reaching every part of your body. Then, slowly and gently, release the air through your mouth.

How do you feel? Do you feel any difference in your body or emotions? Full breathing allows not only a healthy body but also a calmer mind and more stable emotions, as well as healthy and vital cells that will forge your daily energy.

This concept of breathing is so broad that we could develop it in several books. But our goal is to give you tools to help you in a practical way to connect with your body, with health and with holistic wellness. That is why we would like to ask you this question, *When you feel anger and frustration, how is your breathing? And when you feel peaceful, calm and happy, what is your breathing like?*

Moments of stress generate fast, shortened and shallow breathing (usually called clavicular or "high breathing," which requires our maximum effort to obtain very little air). The body prepares itself to face a particular danger, charging itself with adrenaline to save our lives in the face of an unknown threat.

The problem is that the stress that helps the body to overcome moments of crisis should only last a few minutes, no more. Because when stress spreads, it is no longer favorable and becomes counterproductive. In addition, when stress hormones are "turned on" to help the body overcome this moment of threat, our **growth system** (which is in charge of making our organism grow under optimal conditions) and **immune system** (which protects us from external agents that threaten our health, such as viruses and bacteria) are "closed off," to use all available energy against the perceived danger.

A body under constant stress causes cells to age and die faster, impoverishing the functions of our entire organism.

Hydration

Today we all know that our body is mostly water (73% to be exact) and to be healthy, we all *should* drink two liters of water per day. What you may not know is that cells are mostly water, more than 80%. Therefore, by not having enough water, cells die. In addition, water plays a vital role in the cell's formation.

Staying hydrated helps the creation and healthy formation of cells. But there are a number of things you need to know about *good hydration.*

First, the *quantity*. It has been taken as a universal parameter to drink an amount of two liters of water per day. But we need to consider the state and health of the person involved. For example, if there is fluid retention, it is advisable to correct this imbalance before drinking that amount of water. Regarding this famous two liters, there is a **special formula** that is applied according to the weight of each particular person. This formula was created by Frank Suarez, an expert in metabolism.

This formula is as follows: Your weight in ounces divided by sixteen will give you the number of glasses of water of 8 ounces that you should drink per day.

YOUR WEIGHT (ounces) ÷ 16 = Number of Glasses of Water
Example: If you weigh 160, then you should drink
10 glasses of water each day.

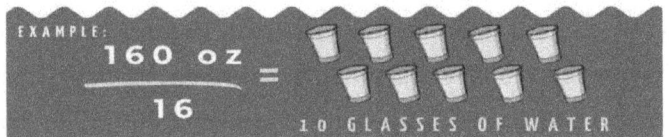

Second, *quality and type*. Drinking water does not mean drinking an infusion, it is not drinking tea, coffee, soda or carbonated water. Water is **water**. You can drink it naturally flavored with lemon, but it must be water.

Many people believe that by drinking liquids throughout the day, several cups of coffee or tea, they are hydrating themselves, but they are NOT.

To keep the body hydrated and for this hydration to reach the cells, our body needs water. Sorry for the insistence. Regarding the quality, drinking tap water is not the same as drinking bottled water or filtered water. The ideal thing is to be able to drink the best quality water you have at hand. If it is bottled, it is more advisable to drink from a glass bottle than from a plastic bottle. Glass containers do not alter the contents or the taste of the liquid. On the contrary, plastic has thousands of carbon chains that, when they begin to disintegrate, are introduced into our bodies every time we drink (according to studies carried out by the World Health Organization).

The Magic Of Hot Water

The last vital detail about water is the *temperature.* It is not the same to drink ice water, natural water, then hot water. According to Ayurveda, Agni (the fire energy present in the metabolism) is located in our stomach. Agni is our transforming force, the digestive fire that controls our metabolism and allows us to absorb the necessary nutrients to preserve our health. The metabolic process is a "cooking" process where food is divided into nutrients and waste and it is a hot procedure. Therefore, all cold drinks or foods we ingest shut down and slow down this digestion process, contributing to metabolic and digestive problems (like heartburn or stomachaches).

https://www.marianandpablo.com/benefits-of-hot-water

Elimination

All cells eliminate waste. The whole process of tissue creation and formation inevitably requires the correct elimination of wastes. If this third step is interrupted in any way by stress, sleep deprivation or bad nutrition, it leads to a lack of energy and eventually to disease. We can breathe more consciously and fully and hydrate better by drinking more water, but how do we help our cells to better eliminate waste? Do you have any idea? It's very simple—with *movement* and, of course, *proper nutrition*.

Physical exercise is vital not only to tone the body. Its main function is to bring health to our whole organism, mainly by helping the cells achieve proper toxins and waste elimination.

If you start respecting these three basic needs of your cells, you will not only feel better, but you will also increase your energy and vitality greatly.

Being happy is simple. The difficult thing is to be simple.

There is another secret and we share it with you now—time is gold. Yes, time is **gold**. The time you spend during the day not only helps you perform different tasks but also allows your body to function in a certain way. Circadian rhythms govern our lives. This means that our life is intrinsically linked to nature and the universe.

For Ayurveda, one of the healthiest habits that we have lost is to *get up at sunrise and go to bed at sunset*. Getting up when the sun rises and going to bed when the sun sets connects our organism with the rhythms of nature.

Remember that your biological rhythms are just that: daily calendars that govern your life according to the natural environment of which you are a central part.

With the access to electric energy, we have forgotten that the night is an important time to rest, not for work or study, and this simple habit generates many imbalances, not only at a mental level, but also at a physical one.

A great Ayurvedic physician, **Dr. Robert Svoboda**, shares his thoughts, "We human beings can make thousands of misalignments in our lives, but the most important habit we lost is the habit of waking up at dawn and going to bed at dusk." When we learn to align ourselves to the natural rhythms of life, our life flows naturally and healthily, effortlessly.

We are now going to share with you two exercises that will help you discover how your energy is today.

EXERCISE 1

This first exercise is very simple. If you want to get a general idea of how your energy is today, we recommend you take the following test. You only have to answer the following questions with *yes* or *no*. To see the final result, you must count 2 points for each *yes* and 0 points for each *no*.

1. Do you concentrate easily?
2. Do you manage to remember words and situations without effort?
3. Do you usually have exciting foods such as tea, chocolate, sugar or coffee?
4. Do you like learning new things?
5. Do you make use of your creativity both at home and at work?
6. Are you productive in your daily tasks?
7. Do you enjoy your social life, meeting new people or having new experiences?
8. Do you usually sleep well at night?
9. Do you wake up with energy?
10. Do temperature changes affect you either physically or emotionally? Do you suffer from allergies, insomnia, etc., during the changing of seasons?

11. Do you enjoy starting new projects?
12. Do you feel you are in control of your emotions in times of conflict or stress?

Results:

From **0 to 9 points**: it would be important that you focus on making a change in your daily routine to achieve the energy you need. Connect with your body, your mind, observe your emotions, review your diet and see if there is anything that you feel needs to be modified. Everything can be transformed to live a better life. If you have any doubts, we advise you to consult a health professional.

From **10 to 14 points**: acceptable. You have energy that oscillates at times. You feel enthusiastic but then you are exhausted. Perhaps in times of stress or conflict, you feel that life is overwhelming. We recommend that you reflect on your daily habits to determine what is draining your energy when you need it to stay healthy and balanced at all times.

From **15 to 20 points**: Very good! You have very good energy. This means that your performance in life is quite good. However, there is always room for improvement. You are following a healthy path and we advise you to keep paying attention to your emotions to identify any moment that may generate unwanted stress. Congratulations!

EXERCISE 2

Here is the second exercise. Keep track of your daily schedule. You can write down in your notebook what time you usually get up in the morning and what time you usually go to sleep. Write down an ideal goal for you. What time would you like your day to start and end? For seven days, you will get up and go to bed **29 minutes earlier** than usual. These numbers are special, so make an effort to respect them. If you usually get up at 10 a.m., then for seven days, you will get up at 9:31 a.m., if you go to bed at 11 p.m. Then for seven days you will do so at 10:29 p.m.

Write down in your notebook how you are feeling. Is there any difference in your thoughts or rest? Remember, every day is a new opportunity to connect with our talents. Take advantage of every minute. Below is a sample chart as an example:

Monday	Tuesday	Wednesday	Thursday	Friday	Saturday	Sunday
6:31 - I feel very tired	6:31 - clearer mind	6:31 - my body feels energized	6:31 - tired but alert	6:31 - energetic and effortless	8:31 - eager to do things	8:31 - cheerful and energetic.

Part 2: Mind

Chapter 4

"The main cause of unhappiness is not the situation,
but your thoughts about the situation."
- Eckhart Tolle

We all have a demon within us. What do we mean? Here we are not talking about religion or superstitious beliefs. We all possess an inner voice that limits us and that works 365 days a year, practically 24 hours a day, every day. To clarify this concept a little, we are going to share a story with you.

The Story of the Wolf

One morning, the old leader of the Cherokee tribe told his grandson about a very difficult battle that rages within each person. "Little one," he told him, "this great battle is between two big, strong wolves. One of them is evil and is made of anger, envy, jealousy, sadness, regret, greed, arrogance, self-indulgence, guilt, resentment, pride, inferiority, lies, false pride, superiority and ego. The other wolf is different. It is made of joy, peace, love, hope, serenity, humility, kindness, goodness, benevolence, friendship, empathy, generosity, truth, compassion and faith."

"And do they fight hard, Grandpa?" the little boy asked.

"Yes, little boy, this battle happens within you, within me and within every person who walks this earth."

> *The grandson, sitting on the grass, looked down from his grandfather's wise eyes and stared at the grass for a while. He meditated for a minute and then asked him, "Which wolf wins, grandfather?"*
>
> *To which the wise old Cherokee replied, "The one you feed."*

This monster reminds us of what we failed at, what we have done wrong—our shortcomings, what we should have done but never did. He disguises himself as our parents' lost hopes, our friends' and peers' expectations and colleagues' criticisms, and a myriad of frustrations and events that have left deep pain and discomfort in our hearts.

This monster dwells in that space inside our mind that only sees the negative in us, the flaws, faults and failings. Nothing else. The bad news is that this monster has made its home inside us and there it will stay until the last day of our lives, it has an irrevocable contract and unlimited lodging. The good news is that we can fight it and finally stop paying attention to it so that its influence no longer affects our life. You probably never heard about this monster's existence and have believed that this voice is your real voice and the only one that exists within you. But it is not you, nor is it the only voice you have.

Do not blame yourself for letting it guide you. Now that you know this, we can begin an action plan to tame the monster.

The first step is always to become aware and realize that this voice is not us. It does not represent us, nor does it represent who we really are. The second step is to feed that second wolf that lives inside us. The good wolf.

Thus we begin to empower ourselves, recognizing who we really are, beings in constant evolution and change. It is vital that you remember this— the bad wolf is not you. This wolf is simply a voice from within us, from our unconscious mind and it just disguises itself as our partner, our colleague, a person at work with whom we do not get along at all, and even family and friends.

It is important to recognize that these voices are internal and that just as they are internal, **they belong to us, although they do not represent us**. And because they belong to us, we can find a way to disarm them.

We all have these inner demons and they have more to do with our belief system than with the reality we live day by day. Therefore, it is essential to understand that the career you have, the family you created, your health and the life you live day by day are not represented by these inner demons.

At some point in our lives, we all wonder if what we are doing is right. There is a phrase that says, "*Perfect is the enemy of Good.*" And yet, why do we want to be perfect? Why do we want everyone to like us? Why do we expect everything to go right on the first try?

Life is a learning experience. And like all learning, it's a process and it takes time. There are times when things go well and times when we learn. There are no good and bad. This voice of good and bad is an inner voice that is not real. You are what you came here to do in this life.

Remember that these internal voices can be disarmed because they do not represent the quality of life you can have.

"The body does not know the difference between an experience and a thought, you can literally change your biology, neurological circuits, chemistry, hormones and genes, simply by having an inner experience."
- Dr. Joe Dispenza

In previous chapters, we talked about your body, the temple of the soul. What are your inner voices saying about your body? What do you usually think about your own body, about your soul temple? Have you ever considered your body as a temple? Have you ever looked at it without paying attention to the "flaws"? Have you ever looked at yourself in the mirror without looking for a flaw but simply to admire the person you are and the beauty in you?

All the faults and flaws are inner voices of our demons, but they do not represent us; they do not represent who we really are. They do not represent you as a whole person in a process of change and constant evolution.

That is why it is important to first detect and become aware of these voices. When a critical or judgmental thought comes to you, or a negative thought arises about yourself, your partner, your family, or about the work you are doing, use this formula that we are going to share with you now to disarm this inner demon.

It is simple and consists of three parts. You only need these three simple steps. Any demon, big or small, can be disarmed. It is a very simple way to tame and disarm this evil wolf that we all have inside us.

EXERCISE

Whenever a hostile or limiting thought appears, you should observe it and then disarm it by answering these three short questions:

1. How much truth is in what I am saying to myself?
2. Is it true/real?
3. Is it really an *absolute* truth?

Becoming aware every time these thoughts appear through these questions allows us to engage in an internal dialogue that **disarms and deactivates limiting beliefs** and our inner demons. In this way, we tame the evil wolf and give way to the good white wolf. As a practical exercise, you can **make a list of recurring dialogues** that you have in your mind.

For example:
"I am good for nothing."
"I always do everything wrong."
"I never do things right."
"I am a failure."
"Life is always against me."
"Nobody loves me."
"I'm worthless."

Then try to answer the three questions we shared a few lines back. *"I am good for nothing."* How much truth is in what I am saying? Am I really good for nothing? Is it true that I am good for nothing? Is it an absolute truth? Is there *nothing* I can do well?

For this to really work and bear fruit, you must perform this exercise on a regular basis. Ideally, every day or every time you notice when a limiting thought appears. This daily exercise will allow you to take away the power of the evil wolf, your personal demon and your inner monster. You will be able to regain and recover your inner power and control of your mind.

This exercise of disarming inner demons is a very profound exercise created by speaker, lecturer and writer **Tony Robbins**. He recommends doing this exercise with total honesty, from the heart, understanding that all inner voices are not ours. They are voices that we have been hearing since we were children or that have come from our parents in some moments of stress, but they do not define us as a person. They do not define us, nor do they define our life path.

Just as in the story of the wise Cherokee grandfather, the quality of our life depends on which wolf we decide to feed. If I deposit my beliefs thinking that I am really good for nothing, then that is the reality that I will be materializing. That is how my life will materialize. If I think that I am really a failure in business, then that is the reality that I will be co-creating with my beliefs and my thoughts.

Every phrase we say to ourselves, every thought we hold as a belief, must be something we feel from the heart. If you really believe that you are a failure and that this is an absolute truth for you, and that is what you will be manifesting in your life.

But if you realize that this thought is not an absolute reality, that it is not true, **then you have found the moment of power**. That is the moment to realize that it is just a thought and that thoughts can be changed. Any thought can be changed.

> *"Selfish is not the one who thinks of himself,*
> *but the one who does not think of others."*
> **- Buddha**

You cannot give what you do not have. That is a bit of a harsh phrase. We all want to help others. Have you ever seen an old lady trying to carry a heavy bag or trying to cross the street? You do not hesitate to go and give her a hand.

Human beings have an innate quality, already installed in our cells, of cooperation. Whenever we can, we will try to help those in need. We are beings of cooperation, not competition, as Charles Darwin once stated. We did not come here to trample each other to reach an imaginary summit. We came here to grow and expand our abilities and to unleash our true potential to do what we came here to be, to fulfill our soul's mission.

But it often happens that we give what we do not yet have. And here, there is an imbalance. **No one can give to another something that they have not given first to themselves**. In the same way, no one should teach others something they have not yet lived and experienced in their own life.

This has nothing to do with selfishness. Following the Buddha's teachings, selfishness is not one who thinks of himself but one who does not think of others. It has to do with a state of coherence. We cannot give advice on something that we have not first tried. Because the most important part of any learning process is experiencing it.

We have experienced great conflicts with other people, especially with family members, which are the ones that hurt the most. At the beginning, we have lived these experiences with great pain. And then came the questions, *Why us? What did we really do to generate this violent reaction in the other person? Why are we going through this situation that is so unfair and so harmful?*

Then we change that "why" to "what." *What is life showing us this for? What do I feel this pain for? What is the purpose? What can I learn from all this?*

And finally, after a long time, many techniques, mentoring and teachings, we understood that the question still had to keep growing in order to arrive at "how." *How do I choose to live this situation? How do I choose to live or experience this pain/anger/etc?*

Today, we feel grateful for everything we have lived through and for all the conflicts and pains. Strange, isn't it? Because even though we have worked through most of these conflicts and have managed to heal them, the greatest transformation came from within ourselves.

For this reason, in these pages, we want to give you something that we have already experienced to help you heal the inner pain that you may carry in your heart.

We have explained that we all have inner demons and that it is important to recognize them, to be able to heal them, and to be able to transform the evil wolf into a good wolf.

To complete this idea a little more, we are going to share with you the myth of Chiron.

> ### The Deepest Pain
>
> *Greek mythology tells that there was once a great centaur named Chiron. Unlike other gods, Chiron was very peaceful, wise and intelligent and liked to spend his days learning about philosophy, music and other arts. One day Heracles (or Hercules) accidentally stabs an arrow covered by Hydra's venom into one of his Chiron's legs. Such is the pain that Chiron felt when he decided to study different arts to find relief and a cure for his tragedy. The hydra's venom possessed a strange curse that prevented the wound from healing completely, and after a while, the pain returned with full force. As Chiron focused all his attention on finding a cure for his ailment, many other gods came to him for medical help. This is how Chiron became the god's physician, using all he had learned in trying to heal his pain to help others.*

The wisdom Chiron had gained in trying to heal himself was now the key to healing others.

Chiron is the archetype of **our deepest pain**, the one that pushes us to look for a cure and also the one that makes us wise to this pain and then helps others to go through their own.

Why are we sharing this story with you? Just like Chiron, we began this path of healing to alleviate our own pain, tame and silence our demons and relieve our own anguish.

Time, experience, practice and also conflicts have made us experts in the healing and self-knowledge field. Our biggest conflict was (and maybe it is for you too) toxic relationships, and especially toxic family relationships.

In this chapter, we shared with you the keys to find a healthier relationship with those inner voices that often turn into demons.

Which wolf do you decide to feed today? If you decide to continue feeding the evil wolf, then remember that all this food that is reaching this wolf will materialize in the form of life experiences. That is, all this anguish, anger and rage will materialize in our material and physical life, affecting our body. There is always time to feed the right wolf. It is never too late. There is always time to listen to these inner voices and disarm them with love and tranquility.

In this part of the book, we offer you to heal your inner demons today. We're going to disarm them and deactivate them, but in a loving way that can give you knowledge, self-perception and a greater awareness of your own inner world.

Chapter 5

*"We must go deep within ourselves,
where we will find the place where our authentic self resides,
and then the secret of happiness will be revealed to us."*
- Dr. Deepak Chopra

Acceptance + responsibility + guilt

Acceptance is not tolerance; acceptance is not tolerating or putting up with life. It is not surrendering to your life events because that is what you are stuck with or because God may have wanted it that way. **Neither God nor the universe wants your grief, your sorrow or your suffering**. Quite the contrary. To better explain these profound concepts, we are going to share with you a short story.

The Gift of the Wise Master

In a very precarious and very quiet temple there was an old master, giving classes on life to a group of disciples. He was known to be a very wise man and it was said among the villagers that he had attained enlightenment.

One day, a man passed by the temple and decided to challenge the master. He was trying to provoke a reaction in the old man and also to feed his ego by proving that he was nothing more than an old crackpot. He decided to barge into one of the classes and confront him. The wise man's disciples protested against the idea, but the old man accepted the challenge.

> *The young man did not take long to vent all his anger and rage by cursing and even spitting at the calm master. He shouted every known insult and offended even his ancestors.*
>
> *For several hours he did everything possible to drive him to any kind of reaction. But the old man remained passive. Already exhausted, the young man left the temple. Disappointed by the fact that their master accepted so many insults and provocations, the young disciples asked him, "Master, how could you let that man say those things to you? Why did you do nothing?"*
>
> *He answered, "If someone comes to you with a gift and you do not accept it, to whom does the gift belong?"*
>
> *"Well, to the one who tried to deliver it." replied one of the disciples.*
>
> *"The same goes for envy, anger and insults," the master added. "When they are not accepted, they continue to belong to the one who carried them."*

If you do not accept that a conflicting event defines you as a person or defines the rest of your life, then you are accepting your power as the creator of your reality, and you do not accept the gift of the event you have experienced. Do you understand?

You are responsible for your life. You. Not your family, not your country, not the government, not your doctor, not your boss. **You are the one** who determines the quality of the life you want to live, and you are responsible for creating it. No one else is.

To stay in a place of guilt is to settle into a victim's role of, *Poor me, look at all that has happened to me, look at all that I suffered, life is so hard on me.* Instead, adopt the thinking that, *Life is mine, it belongs to me, and I will shape it based on my values and beliefs, and based on what I deserve and what I want for myself and for my loved ones.* Notice the difference?

We are always the masters of our own life. Always. There are no external factors that can determine our life and our future. Unless we choose to do so.

Perhaps these words are easy to understand, but putting them into practice is not always so simple. In the case of family, personal relationships, work relationships, etc., we must be aware **that we are the ones who define the experiences**, which is to say, it is never what happens to us, but how we live it.

When it comes to a family relationship, it is important to realize that we cannot control the other person in the same way that we control our own lives or think we do. We are not responsible, much less to blame, for **the perceptions of others**.

One of the most important keys to a healthy relationship is acceptance. To accept the other, as we mentioned before, is not to tolerate them. Accepting a family member, a partner, a boss, etc., means **understanding their history**, both past and present, without judgment or criticism. Judgment and criticism usually ends up bringing about impending doom. **In acceptance, there is a choice.**

What does this mean? That if violence of any kind is expressed in any relationship, you have the power and the responsibility to say, "Enough!" You have the power to hinder the anger or pain that a person has created. You can accept that this is their reality, but refuse to let it be a part of yours.

Let's make something crystal clear—acceptance is not resignation, nor is it accepting or approving of something that hurts us. On the contrary, acceptance gives us the freedom to see the other person with loving, non-judgmental eyes.

To accept a person is to love all parts of him or her, even though we may not entirely agree with everything. To accept the other is to accept myself. Let us remember that we cannot give to others what we do not give ourselves first.

What are your thoughts usually like when you look in the mirror? What do you think when you see your body in the mirror while trying on new clothes? **Acceptance means to love**, to appreciate lovingly, to understand and embrace fully as it is, not as we would like it to be.

The Power Of Opinion

To address the following topic we are going to tell you a brief story that happened to us a few years ago. A friend of ours posted on Facebook the following question: How *much Paracetamol should I give my one-year-old baby who is running a fever?*

From our Ayurveda knowledge, following a natural path, we replied, *You could try a pinch of fresh or powdered ginger, which can help lower the temperature and strengthen the immune system.*

What happened next left us stunned and confused. We began to receive violent responses, insults and even threats for our thoughtlessness in giving this advice. This taught us several things: first, not to interfere in another person's learning process. And second, not to intervene when we are not asked to do so.

A great friend once told us, "It's never what one says, but what the other person hears." Therefore, the opinion, however loving it may be, if it is not asked for, only **gets in the way and interferes** with the natural process of each person's growth.

> "It is never what one says, but what the other person hears."

When we give our opinion, there is usually a presupposition but not a certainty of fact. This means that our mind creates a hypothesis of what might be happening if it were to happen. Before presupposing, it is more important **to ask**. When we ask, we give space for the other person to be able to express themselves freely, avoiding pre-judgment. If, beyond all this, you decide to share your opinion with someone, you should know that you will have to take responsibility for the consequences. **An opinion can be condemning.**

We live in a very sensitive time where everything is judged, criticized and canceled. When someone makes a mistake, it is often exposed and labeled as out of line and almost a crime. With these words, we do not mean to endorse any type of inappropriate behavior, but rather to refer to our own thoughts regarding the actions of others.

Let us use a real example to be a little clearer. For a while, we lived across the street from a woman named Monica, who was very loving to animals, but not so much to people.

One day a young couple moves in near her house. The next day, when we saw her at the bakery, she told us, "Did you see that we have new neighbors? They seem strange. I am sure they do witchcraft. The woman is surely a witch because I saw her with a red scarf on her head, tied in a knot. That is what witches do. So just to be safe, don't go near them to avoid her doing something bad to you."

Monica is not a bad person, but her opinion about the new neighbors has not helped her—quite the contrary. By freely dishing out her conjectures about these strangers, she not only ruined something that could have been a nice relationship with these people, but also began to make her lifelong neighbors uncomfortable. She began to spend more time alone because of her insistent criticism and judgment.

The dangerous thing about an opinion is that with enough insistence, **it becomes a certainty** for the person who holds it, and a certainty **then becomes a belief. Beliefs are the builders of our reality.**

If we believe that life is hard, then our life will be full of obstacles and difficulties because that is how we have designed it within ourselves. That is how we manifest it to the outside world. Therefore, think twice before creating an opinion about something or someone because it may be creating an unfavorable reality for you.

These thoughts we have are ways of feeding the demons we keep inside us. Remember, which wolf are you feeding today? **A thought grows in certainty and graduates into a belief.** And it is this belief that determines the picture of life you will see every day.

Beliefs are the builders of our reality.

EXERCISE

We are now going to teach you a way to manage pain with a practical exercise. This exercise was created by Dr. Deepak Chopra and explained in his book *Synchrodestiny*.

Today we are going to teach **you how to manage your pain**. This exercise requires only 10 minutes of your time. Ready?

STEP 1

Find a place where you can sit quietly and undisturbed. You will begin by meditating for a few minutes (if you have never meditated or if you wish to have a guide, go to the following link: https://www.marianandpablo.com/gratitude-guided-meditation).

You can take a few deep breaths to find that calm space inside you, with your eyes closed.

STEP 2

Think of **an event or situation** in the past that upset you. It can be an argument, a conflict, or a time when your feelings were hurt.

STEP 3

Once you have placed yourself at that point in time, try to recall this moment focusing on **all the details possible** (such as moment of day, weather, the clothes you were wearing, etc.). Try to remember and recall all the details of that discussion, that moment of stress and conflict. **Make a mental movie** of exactly what happened.

The first step in dealing with pain is to **identify exactly what you are feeling**—is it just anger or is it something else? Which word best describes what you are feeling regarding this memory?

STEP 4

Find a word that encompasses what you are feeling. Your best description of this painful memory, and concentrate on that word for a few seconds.

STEP 5

Let your attention gradually shift from that word to your body. What **physical sensations** do you feel as a result of reliving this memory? All emotions have inseparable mental and physical aspects. *Feelings occur in the mind and in the body at the same time.*

STEP 6

Perceive the sensations that have originated this event you are thinking about: Are your hands tense? Do you feel any pressure in your stomach? Is there any part of your body that hurts? **Perceive the physical experience** of this emotion and **locate it** in a specific point of your body.

STEP 7

The next step is to **express the feeling**. Place your hand on the part of the body where you feel it is located and say out loud, "It hurts here." If the pain has more than one location, touch each part and repeat the phrase, "It hurts here."

Within us we have the power to make the pain of any pain, any anguish or conflict disappear. Our reactions to external events are located in the body. We create emotions that generate physical pain.

When we understand this simple fact, we can learn to change the way we respond to external events. **We can choose** our reaction to events. If we react with anger, rage, hostility, depression, anxiety or some other intense emotion, our bodies follow that direction and create hormones secretion, muscle contractions and other related physical reactions that produce pain.

Feelings occur in the mind and in the body at the same time. We create emotions that generate physical pain.

We must always keep in mind that these effects are our responsibility because we have the capacity and the power to modify our reactions and make them less harmful. **We have the power to heal ourselves**. We are capable of freeing ourselves from drama and emotional turbulence. Meditate for a few minutes on the concept of the **personal responsibility** you have for any emotional reaction.

STEP 8

Once you locate and recognize the pain and once you have taken responsibility for your existence, **you can release it**. Place your attention on the part of the body where you feel the pain. With each exhalation, release that tension you are holding. Focus for half a minute on releasing the tension and pain in your body with each breath, releasing the air through your mouth. Let it out, let it go. Breathe it out. Get it out of your body.

You have the power to heal yourself.

STEP 9

The next step is to **share the pain**. Imagine that you could talk to the person involved in the situation you have remembered for this exercise. What would you say to this person?

Remember that this person was not the real cause of your pain. You had the emotional reaction that manifested itself in your physical pain. *But you have taken responsibility*. And with this in mind, what would you say to this person?

Whatever you decide to say to them will be unique to you and your situation. Whatever you say to share the pain you felt will help you to **eliminate this experience from your consciousness forever** because you will have already *transformed* it. It will cease to be a traumatic experience and become a healthy experience, a transformed experience. Share what you felt and what you feel now and how you plan to handle these feelings in your future.

IMPORTANT NOTE: You do not need to actually talk to this person. You can simply write what you would say to him or her in your notebook as a letter. Being able to "get the words out of your body" and onto paper is a great emotional cleansing exercise.

STEP 10 (Optional)

To finish releasing these dense emotions, you can take the written letter and set it on fire (minding the place and being extra careful when lighting the paper). Then, take a moment to observe as the flames engulf the paper, changing its color and finally consuming any evidence of it ever existing. In the same way, this pain would have vanished from your body and your mind.

Whenever you feel any emotional turbulence, whenever you feel that your emotions are unbalanced, you can do this exercise. When you have finished it, take a moment to celebrate that this painful experience has been transformed and has served you to transcend to a higher level of consciousness. Remember that transformation entails transcendence. Doing this exercise implies that you have taken a step up in your level of consciousness.

If you practice it regularly, you will eventually be able to free yourself completely from any pain and emotional turbulence and clear the way to experience healthier emotions and a lighter inner world.

https://www.marianandpablo.com/how-to-manage-pain-exercise

Transformation brings transcendence.

Chapter 6

"All personal breakthroughs begin with a belief change."
- Tony Robbins

In order to change that which harms or limits you, you must **return to the starting point**. This means that you must create a new beginning in your life.

If today were the first day of a new life, what would you do? What would you have for breakfast? What would you wear? What would you say to yourself when you look in the mirror?

First, we must get rid of what no longer serves us. We must make room within ourselves to make room for everything new.

Ho'oponopono, an ancient art of forgiveness, teaches that everything we desire can be materialized to become part of our reality. But first, we must let go of all the **toxic garbage** we have inside us. The aim of **Ho'oponopono** is to discover who we really are, beyond our own judgment, the judgment of others and what we have believed about ourselves up to now.

Ho'oponopono means *to correct a mistake, to rectify a mistake*, to correct something that is wrong, or to amend something that is not correct. In Hawaiian, *"ho"* means *"cause,"* and *"pono"* means *"perfection."* In other words, what we seek is to find perfection through correcting an error that may be translated into the form of limiting beliefs and thoughts.

Ho'oponopono helps us clear blockages and memories that generate painful beliefs within us. With Ho'oponopono, we seek inner peace, cleansing our inner self of any negativity that may be generating internal or external pain.

The aim of Ho'oponopono is to discover who we really are, beyond our own judgment, the judgment of others, and beyond what we have believed about ourselves up to now.

We have already mentioned above how much our opinions and thoughts, these inner demons, can affect us. All human beings live by systematically repeating toxic, limiting thoughts, mental patterns and negative emotions.

This accumulation of information is what Ho'oponopono calls **memories** and can come from ancestors, early childhood experiences and our adult life development.

According to Morrnah Simeona, a former Ho'oponopono master and guide, "We are the sum total of our experiences, which is to say that we are burdened by our pasts. When we experience stress or fear in our lives, if we look carefully, we will find that the cause is actually a memory. It is the emotions which are tied to these memories which affect us now."

That is why it is so important to bring the thoughts we have on a daily basis to our awareness. Are they really ours? Do they belong to us? Did we create them, or are we inheriting them generation after generation?

These thoughts generate a **belief system** whose power is to create the physical reality you experience every day. Is the body you have today the body you always dreamed of or is it the body you criticize every day?

There is an ancient Vedic proverb that goes like this, *"If you want to know what your thoughts were like yesterday, look at your body today. And if you want to know what your body will be like tomorrow, look at your thoughts today."*

It is very important to understand that our body is nothing more than a vibrational manifestation of our inner energy. We have said that we are created through the five elemental forces of the universe: ether, air, fire, water and earth. And these forces are vibrations of matter that create everything that exists. They have to do with a vibration. And this vibration is also seen through the **thoughts** we have every day, our **emotions,** and above all, our **beliefs**. Thoughts that have become certainties, that we take as absolute truths. These beliefs create the reality we live in today.

> *"If you want to know what your thoughts were like yesterday, look at your body today. And if you want to know what your body will be like tomorrow, look at your thoughts today."*
>
> **- Ayurvedic proverb**

So we ask you again, *What is your body like today? What is your life like today? What do you think your life is like? And what would it be like if you were to start a new life today?*

We are creators of the chaos in which we live. This sentence may be a bit strong, and you may feel it is not quite true. And it may not be true for you. However, everything you experience today is the result of the thoughts and beliefs that exist within you. Yes, even pain, illness and trauma. We know that it is difficult to understand that we have **created this**.

It is essential to understand that nothing has been created with the intention of being unhappy, but that this toxic accumulation of beliefs is housed in our unconscious mind and it is from here that we create the reality we live.

This is why it is so important to become aware of the importance of feeding the right wolf. If we are consciously feeding the good wolf, the wolf generates abundance, health and well-being. A calm wolf, a wolf that keeps us in the right path of self-love, respecting others and cherishing the beauty in life.

According to Ho'oponopono, we all have things to heal. We all have memories to cleanse, to erase, to remove from our consciousness. And these memories are lodged in the deepest corners of our **subconscious mind**. That is where our inner child dwells. Our inner child does not judge or criticize and accepts all beliefs as absolute truths. It recreates them in our lives, generating patterns of thought and action.

We all have thousands of thoughts a day. According to scientific studies, it is estimated that we have about **60,000 thoughts a day,** every day. This is not a problem. The problem is that the vast majority of those thoughts that we have, and here you should pay close attention to, **are negative and an almost exact replica** of the previous day.

And if that was not enough, they are not even ours! Did you know that? It sounds unbelievable, but that is how it is. Most of our thoughts today are repetitions of the previous day and the day before that and so on. When analyzing them, you can detect that even these thoughts are not your own, but are replicas of things you have been hearing throughout your life and in your childhood (especially from birth to six years old), which is when you absorb everything you see and feel around you and with what you then generate **your mental programming.**

In our early childhood, everything we see and experience will become the program for the rest of our lives. Everything we experience will create a belief within us that will later on create the reality we live in.

The great doctor of Cell Biology, Bruce Lipton, talks a lot about this process in his book *The Biology of Belief.* Many of the beliefs that will create our reality will not even be ours, but we will adopt the beliefs of our parents (as they have adopted the beliefs of their parents) to create a picture of reality.

To give you an example, one day, in line at a bank, a woman decided to set down her heavy purse on the floor. The lady behind her said, "No! Do not do that, you will lose your money!"

To which the woman replied, "Oh, you are right; it costs so much to earn it." And she put the heavy purse back on her shoulder.

This example we shared with you may or may not feel familiar to you, but there is more than one thing worth mentioning.

The first is that money has no legs and will not go anywhere you do not want it to. So this fear that money "runs away" is not only simple superstition, but it is a belief that has been anchored in our unconscious mind, making us believe it is true.

The second thing we want you to look at is the woman's response. Do you notice something strange? Does it sound familiar? Do you feel that she is wrong in saying what she said? Well, here is the truth: whether money is hard to earn or not hard to earn, reflects your relationship with abundance and your financial situation. It mirrors your **belief about material resources**. If you manage to have money or if it is difficult to earn it, it has to do with your belief, not with a universal reality.

"Whether you think you can or you think you cannot, you are right."
- Henry Ford

This quote from Henry Ford follows just that—it is your belief, not the facts, that determines your experience. It is never what happens to you, but how you choose to experience it. The problem is that most of the time, we unconsciously choose to live out situations through old programming, which is obsolete and no longer useful for our wellbeing in general.

It's never what happens to you, but how you choose to live it.

In the example above, the woman chose to remain uncomfortable, perhaps even hurting her shoulder, rather than put her purse down for fear that her money might disappear.

It is easier to believe that money mysteriously disappears from our purses, maybe running away to a new life, than to take responsibility for our own finances. But the reality is that everything that happens to us not only happens for a reason we do not know about, but we are the creators of that reality. Therefore, if there is something we do not like or something that makes us uncomfortable, we can *change* it.

We will now share with you another story that demonstrates how complex the conditioning of our own beliefs is. This happened in an intensive seminar conducted by T. Harv Eker, a renowned author and businessman.

Stephen had no problem generating money, only keeping it. He was making over $800,000 a year. But just as he was making it, he was losing it. It evaporated. During the seminar, Stephen confessed that as a child, his mother always said, "Rich people are greedy and mean. You should have just enough to live on. If you have more, you are a pig and a bad person."

It's not hard to deduce that his difficulty holding on to money was an unconscious way of continuing to do what his mother had implanted in his mind. Unconsciously, he just wanted to make his mother happy. What kid does not want that?

We are fully free to correct what hurts us, makes us uncomfortable or bothers us. Being happy is a *choice*, not a reward. So use your thoughts, not to condemn yourself and to suffer, but to heal whatever it is you need to heal, to drive you to where you want to go and to achieve what you want to achieve.

Being happy is a decision, not a reward.

Our entire belief system resides within our inner child, in our unconscious mind. And it is there that we have been feeding this inner child with negative beliefs, creating inner demons.

What are the poisons in your life? Surely when reading this question, several situations have come to your mind, even people that have generated damage and pain in your life. It is important for you to know **that nothing happens to hurt you.**

Your inner child is not weaving these beliefs to harm you and to hurt you, but so that you can finally recognize them as your own and release them, clean them and clear the space within you so that you can heal your relationship with yourself.

Everything in life is a learning experience and has come at the perfect time for you to transcend it. Forgive yourself for getting angry or upset, even for taking it out on people who had nothing to do with it, even your pet who came running to you when you were angry, and you pushed him or her away. Then, be grateful for what has happened because it has allowed you to open your eyes and become aware of this situation. When you can project yourself, you can see reality more clearly.

There is a very beautiful phrase, "*Worried about a leaf, you will miss the tree; worried about the tree, you will miss the whole forest.*" This phrase demonstrates that when your focus is on one thing, you miss the big picture and you become distressed because you cannot change a painful situation.

All things happen at the perfect time to help us expand our awareness, open our hearts and overcome any obstacle in our life.

Every pain is also a learning experience. In Ayurveda, we talk about the five **Kleshas**. *Klesha* is a Sanskrit word that means "*poison*" and refers to the poisons that we tend to take, which prevent us from being who we truly are and, above all, from being happy.

Therefore, we must understand that life only brings us learning experiences and understanding, not torments, and that everything that we do not like in our life is there to be corrected, amended and transformed.

We can learn about these five poisons that allow us to understand how the universe works and how we can begin to act without generating unnecessary pain.

In the words of the Buddha, "Pain is inevitable, but suffering is optional." This means that pain is part of life.

If we stub our toe on a piece of furniture in our house (something we have all experienced at one time or another), we focus our attention there (what can be more painful, right?). Then, we realize that perhaps we were distracted and this pain showed us that we should have paid more attention to where we were walking. But if I complain about this pain and the next day I tell my coworkers, I complain to my partner, I get angry with my children, etc., then that pain turns into suffering because I am choosing to focus on the pain instead of the learning.

We are all responsible for our own learning. No one harms us. Life brings us different experiences in order to achieve **a new level of consciousness.**

We mentioned before the concept of your inner child. This notion is also part of psychoanalysis and refers to **all the experiences we have had and that we have been keeping** since we were kids. When we grow up and become structured as adults and independent persons, we learn values, rules, and limits. We also learn how to behave, how to interact with others, how to express love and our needs.

Actually, this concept of the inner child comes from Ho'oponopono, where it is called *Unihipili*. This Unihipili is the deepest part of our beings, the one that houses memories and beliefs. All the information that we have received from the womb and that we have been collecting from our family experience, our ancestors.

Our inner child houses our most sensitive parts, our softest parts.

Maybe you think that healing your inner child is difficult, or maybe you do not know how to connect with your unconscious mind, with your deepest parts. In this chapter, we are going to tell you how to do it in a simple and easy way, but first, we are going to share a personal story from Mariana.

> ### *My moment of awakening*
>
> *Often, "insight" moments come from moments of crisis. And so it was for me. I was at a time in my life when I was very stressed with a lot of work. I was happy with what I was doing, but very sad because I was living in a very conflictive situation with my family. I did not feel that I could connect lovingly with my parents and my brother. I felt that there was a lot of criticism, judgment and even mistreatment. And I felt so much pain and sorrow that I tried to fill all the free spaces in my life with more work so that I could be at home as little as possible. The pain of criticism and judgment was so great that I preferred to be away from home than to spend time with my family.*
>
> *One day I received a message from a good friend of mine inviting me to a cooking course the next Sunday morning. I thought, "I can spend the day at home, enduring the bad treatment and anguish, or I can go and spend my time with other people. Maybe I can even make new friends. And most importantly, I am also going to be able to be with my friend, who I already know and trust." So that day I put on some nice comfortable clothes and walked to catch the train to the cooking class.*
>
> *As I walked, several thoughts filled my mind. I thought about how sad I felt. The helplessness I felt every day at home. What could I do to make my family happy? Then I began to answer my own question. My Dad wants me to finish my degree and get a job. I already had a job (more than one, actually), but my Dad would be happy if I finished my degree. I am going to finish it so he will be happy. My Mom would be happy for me to get married,*

so it would be nice if I could meet somebody nice and get married. Maybe later, she would not be satisfied, and she wants me to have children. Then I should have kids so my parents can be grandparents and be happy. My brother was very angry about my last boyfriend. Maybe I should let my brother choose for me the partner he would accept or consult him if he is okay with the next person coming into my life. But this is almost absurd.

As I pondered all this, I realized that this was never going to be enough, and that I was always going to need something else to make others happy. I came to a conclusion and a hard truth—I would never be able to make my family happy. There was no possibility in the universe to make them happy and for this happiness to be true and lasting. But there was something I could do; there was one happiness that was in my control—mine. I could make myself happy. I could start focusing on my happiness. It was really the only true happiness. Trying to make other people happy was not going to work and, worse, I would devote my whole life to conforming others to no avail.

I realized that happiness is not something to be achieved, not something to be given away, not something to be bought, but something to be experienced and lived within each person.

It was not easy for me to arrive at this truth. I walked around crying when I realized that I could not make my family happy. But I also felt liberated because as much as it hurt to arrive at this truth, I had also found a new truth—I could be happy. No one was stopping me from being happy. Because if my only task in this life was to be happy, then the task was in my hands. To be happy was not something far away, but was actually in my hands, under my own decision and will. I simply had to set my mind to it.

That day I set out to be happy. I recognized that the only thing I needed to be happy was to set my mind to it. And I said to myself, "**Today is the first day of my life.** From today, my life begins because, from today, I start to be

> *happy. And I am going to do everything in my power to be able to find my own happiness, beyond the work I am doing, beyond my family, my career, etc. No one in the world can make me happy except myself. From now on, that is my only task and my only responsibility. Many, many things in our lives can cause us pain, but anchoring ourselves in suffering is a choice."*
>
> *That day I decided to let go of my pain and to start taking care of my own happiness. Today is the first day of my life. From today I will start to be happy.*

With this story, we want to share with you a life vision. Mariana had been trying to fulfill other people's expectations and beliefs. And when she realized that all she wanted in life was to be happy, everything in her life fell into place. She realized that it was much easier to take care of her happiness than to try to make others happy. Because there is no way to make others happy. Happiness is something you share, not something you buy or achieve. Happiness is something personal, not something external. Happiness is a state of mind, not a goal to be achieved.

There is nothing better than to be happy and to see that your family is happy to see you happy. This is the best way to heal a family relationship. That was the best way Mariana found to be able to do something really nice for her family. She found her happiness and was able to share it with others.

Happiness is a state of mind, not a goal to be achieved. Happiness is in the journey, not the destination.

EXERCISE 1

We recommend the following exercise—know your inner child. We mentioned that the inner child is the one that keeps all the accumulation of beliefs and values, both personal and family and transcendental.

Look for a photo of yourself when you were an infant, when you were a little boy or girl. Why do we do this? It is important that you have a photo of yourself when you were a child in your hands and that you take a good look at your photo. Could you get mad at a child like that? Could you really hurt someone like that as a child? You couldn't, right? The problem is that you do. We all do it every day with thoughts, beliefs, and inner dialogues with our demons and evil wolves. That is why, by looking at your picture, you can meet the person who truly gets hurt every time. Your inner child is the one who always gets hurt.

Every step you take in this book allows you to give a little love to that little boy in you and what you see there in the picture. The more love it receives, the better it will do its job of clearing memories to create new, more productive and healthier beliefs.

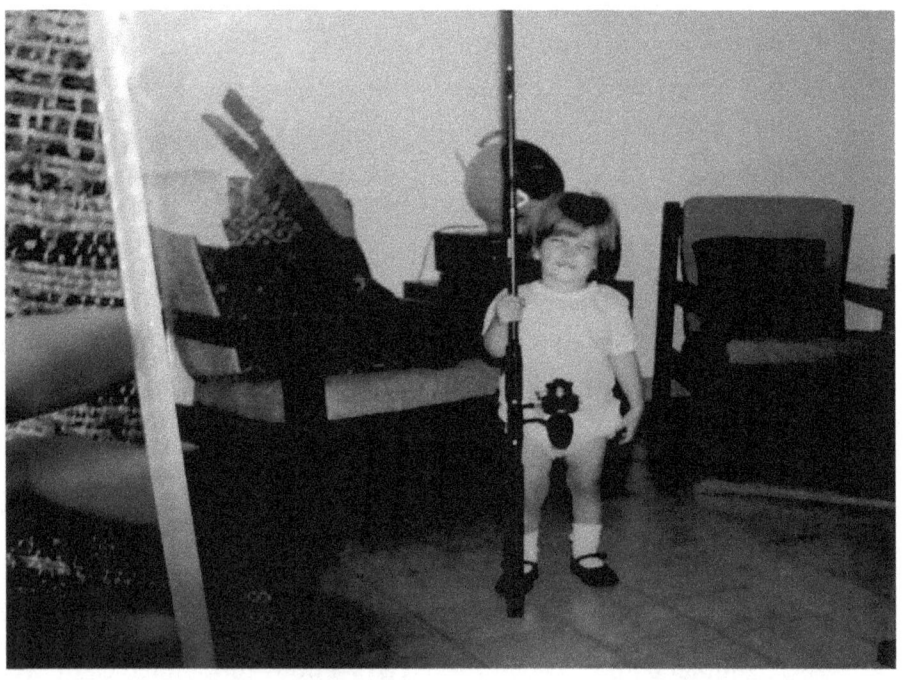

Little Mariana (age 2)

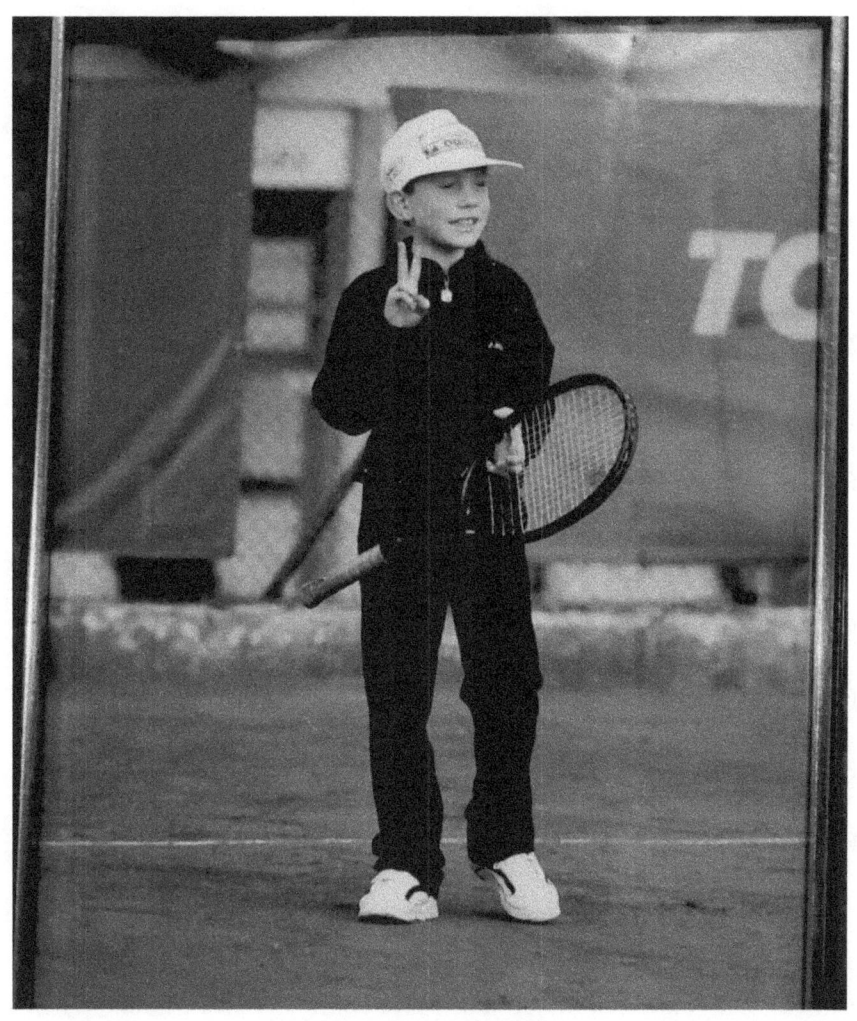

Little Pablo (age 9)

EXERCISE 2

Here's a second practical exercise created by Dean Graziosi, a great speaker, entrepreneur and author. He calls it "The Clarity Tool." Here is what you are going to do:

Think of an affirmation about yourself. Think about what you want to achieve in your life. Write this affirmation of what you want in your life on a piece of paper, and then ask yourself why. Mariana, for example, wanted to be happy. So the question would be, *Why did she wish to be happy?* Once you answer the question, ask yourself again, "Why?" By asking *why* seven times, you will achieve **seven levels of depth** to get to the deepest answer, the one you hide inside you.

Below you will find a guide to help you. We used a simple example of "becoming successful" as our focus.

LEVEL 1: What is important to you about (becoming successful)?

LEVEL 2: Why is it important to you?

LEVEL 3: Why is it important to you?

LEVEL 4: Why is it important to you?

LEVEL 5: Why is it important to you?

LEVEL 6: Specifically, why is it important to you?

LEVEL 7: Why is it important to you?

Mariana came to the conclusion that she wanted to be happy because happiness, in the end, was all she longed for. There were no diplomas, no certificates, no partners, no job that could define her as a person. When she came to this conclusion, she realized that she had value as a person, nothing external added value to her. Her value was within herself.

With this exercise of the seven levels of depth, we propose you write down that goal you want to achieve in this life. What is it that you really want to transform in your life? And ask yourself seven times, *why?* Try to reach deeper levels of knowledge.

Maybe you want a better salary. Why do you want a better salary? Maybe you feel you do not have the salary you deserve. Why do you think you do not have the salary you deserve? Maybe it is because you feel you are overworked. Why do you think you are overworked? Maybe it is because you feel you are worth much more than you are paid. And why do you feel that way? Maybe it is because you work to be valued, but no one values you. Maybe it is because you are not yet giving yourself the value you truly deserve. Notice how deep a question goes. All we really want in life is to be loved, valued, respected, and respected.

What do you want to transform today?

7 levels of depth exercise:
https://www.marianandpablo.com/your-true-why

Part 3: Spirit

Chapter 7

The biggest obstacle to achieving success in what we dream about are the limitations programmed in the subconscious mind.
- Dr. Bruce Lipton

We begin this chapter with a story of an extremely warm and generous person, whom we will call "A." At a family meeting, A made reference to her lack of faith for a specific reason—God's failures. The cause of her lack of faith in God was simple. She explained that if something as important as teeth, indispensable for human survival, are crooked, then it cannot be the work of an intelligent, conscious being, God or whatever one wants to call it simply cannot exist.

We listened carefully to the story and saw how such simple reasoning can justify the lack of faith in an intelligent, conscious universe and a belief in chaos.

According to A's theory, we are here by pure chance and survive by luck. Everything is left to chance. There is no order or guidance, much less a loving entity that takes care of us. The reality is that we could not help but feel sorry and surprised that this simple detail can serve as an excuse to live in mistrust and lack of faith. Everyone is free to think and feel whatever they want about God, the Universe, etc., but to reach the conclusion of a lack of order because of a human characteristic is just unimaginable.

Many people think that when things are different from what one thinks or believes life should be, then there is a fault. God has made a mistake—the universe is flawed.

"It cannot be that a person who has crooked teeth was created in this life to be happy. A person with crooked teeth reflects the belief that life is chaos and that there is no creative force and higher intelligence to keep us alive," A stated with a frown.

Unbelievable, isn't it? But these are thoughts. That is the magic of it all. These thoughts may or may not be your own, but they are thoughts nonetheless, and thoughts can be changed.

The problem with these thoughts is that when they hold on to an opinion, they create a certainty and grow into a belief. These beliefs, of which we have already spoken, are the ones that manifest the creative power of our life, which creates our life experiences day by day.

That is why it is so important to consciously observe the opinions we have of the world. Are they real? Are they absolute truths? If they are not, if there is a tiny drop of doubt, then this means that, most probably, this opinion or this thought is not real and may very well not be our own.

It is likely that these criticisms of life do not even belong to us. Perhaps they are more of a family tradition than a certainty of something we feel in our hearts. And this is what we are going to focus on in this chapter: **the certainties of the heart**, because many times we give a lot of importance to our mind, to our rational part, to reason.

How could it be that God exists if there are people with crooked teeth?

Some people find incredible the possibility that there is a God, that there is a force, a pure and creative consciousness of all matter when there are people with crooked teeth. For many people, disorder or chaos should not exist. In the work environment, disorder or chaos are also taken as capital sins.

It is very difficult to live and coexist in a loving world if we are not able to accept the different perceptions of reality.

Earlier, we talked about the importance of the transforming fire (*Agni*) that is also present in our sense of sight. Let us understand **that every time we see something around us, we are transforming it and it is transforming us as well.**

The mental image we have of life does not represent life itself, it is not the real thing; it is an expectation; it is what we think it should be; it is what we assume life to be because it is based on a set of values, beliefs, thoughts, and traditions that have little to do with real life and much to do with what we expect from life.

Are you a spiritual person and do you feel a connection to your spiritual world? This has nothing to do with the religion you profess. The important thing is to understand that the entire creative force of the universe wants nothing more than our happiness. Having a spiritual world implies trusting life and not so much from the mind, but from the heart. In the same way, any deep transformation in your life should not only happen in your mind, but also in your heart.

It is very difficult to live and coexist in a loving world if we are not able to accept the different perceptions of reality.

Many times, when we make a change in our lives, such as starting a new diet or a new activity, we expect the environment to accompany us. But in reality, it does not work that way.

An essential key to wellness and healing is to **let go of expectations**, and there are many reasons why **expectations are more harmful than kind to us**. For one thing, having too many expectations locks us into what we wish would happen, into thought, into the mental world. Having expectations is not bad, but it is important to understand and learn to realize that we must let go of them at some point—sooner rather than later.

For example, we may wish to buy the house of our dreams or to be congratulated for the presentation we made in our work, or that our child gets a good grade in the exam he/she took at school. But if we cling to these desires, they are no longer just desires, they are expectations, strong longings to live that reality that we imagine. This can cause us great harm, because it does not allow us to accept reality as it is, but leaves us in a state of frustration if things do not happen as we have imagined them in our mind.

As Dr. Deepak Chopra explains in his great book, *The Seven Spiritual Laws of Success*, there are two very important laws that we must respect if we want to live in harmony with the universe and that apply to what we are explaining here. One is the **Law of Detachment**, the other, we are going to save for later.

The law of detachment is based on the belief that in order to achieve anything we desire in life, it is necessary to **renounce the attachment** we have to it. Why? Because attachment to our desires **generates fear and insecurity within us**.

When we relinquish our attachment to our desire, we set it free and connect with trust and the true unlimited creative power of the universe.

When we cling to our expectations, wanting things to happen the way we want them to happen and for others to act the way we believe is right, we are breaking this law because we do not allow life to manifest naturally—we want **to control** the events of our life. But this is not how life truly works.

And here is a magic formula we want to share with you: **happiness is proportional to our level of acceptance and inversely proportional to our expectations**. By this we mean that acceptance gives us the freedom to live life as it is—perfect. Expectations, on the other hand, are anticipations based on subjective constructs in our minds and bind us to a fictitious reality.

Heartfulness

Mindfulness is a trend that has become very well-known lately. This meditation technique focuses on paying attention to the present moment, and observing what is happening with interest, curiosity and acceptance (similar to how a child views the world). Here we do not enter judgment or criticism, but admiration of what we live, as when we were children and looked at the world around us, feeling that everything was new, bright, full of life, mysteries to be solved and challenges to be conquered.

Happiness is proportional to our level of acceptance and inversely proportional to our expectations.

When we grow up and reach adulthood, we leave this curious look at life and turn it into a more discriminating, critical and judgmental look. We classify reality between what is right and what is wrong according to our beliefs and values system, and we discard those things that do not adapt to our desires or interests.

And in this way, **we separate ourselves from the world.** *I want this and nothing else.* This thought, which manifests from our subconscious mind, from our inner child, separates us from the environment. We think, *I am this and the rest is something else.* We endure a constant struggle between our inner world and the inner world of others, which is strange and unrelated to us. The thing about this is that we unconsciously begin to spend more time inside ourselves than outside, isolating ourselves from reality. We start to live in our mind, where everything is controlled, ordered, and adjusted to our tastes and desires.

This process is called **fugue neurosis** and occurs when we disconnect from reality, thinking about past or future events, without paying attention to what we are living in the present moment.

Do not panic; this is completely normal and happens every day because we are afraid that something that happened to us will happen again. Maybe we feel that we have somehow failed and we are dreading going through the same pain. This constant fear of not repeating a pain from the past keeps us in the past and does not allow us to be connected with the present moment.

How many times have we been afraid of meeting new people or starting a new relationship in order to avoid reliving a painful experience from the past? How many people have said, "All men are the same" or "All women are the same"? How many times do we find ourselves in the present repeating stories from the past? How many times do we think that all people are just the same as the person who hurt us before? We even imagine that this completely strange person is going to hurt us just like a previous one did.

The mind takes a step into the future, imagining fantasies, creating unreal worlds of how deeply we are going to hurt and suffer. This is something completely normal. It is a process we all go through, especially in the most important moments of our lives.

Let's take pregnancy as an example. A pregnancy takes nine months of gestation. In these nine months, beyond the medical controls and ultrasounds, we do not have an exact certainty of what is happening inside the body. Then, the mind takes the spotlight, grabs the mike and starts telling us about all the *bad* things that *could* be happening inside the womb. And the anxiety levels rocket to the roof. "Be careful! Do not eat too much of this, you could hurt your baby." "Watch out with this exercise! It could be hurting your baby." "Be careful! You Do not know if the baby is having a bad time." "Maybe he (she) is suffering inside you, and you have not noticed."

We salute mothers all over the world for going through this incredible job of bringing new life to the world. Mothers have the power to connect the immaterial to the material world, summoning a new soul to its material temple. Way to go, mothers!

All these negative thoughts are nothing but those thoughts whispered within us by these voices we call inner demons. It is the evil wolf speaking—a wolf fed with negativity, doubt and fear. It is important to know and remember that fear is the opposite of love, not hate.

Love is an energy that allows transformation and change. Fear is an energy that generates stagnation and paralysis. Fear does not allow us to grow. It leaves us anchored in a state of total immaturity and involution, while love is the energy that allows us to take the leap of faith, to risk it, to take a challenge, conquer our fears, attain our goals and reach the summit of all our dreams.

Love is an energy that allows transformation and change. Fear is an energy that generates stagnation and paralysis.

The fugue neurosis generates **a disconnection between our mind and our heart.** This is the biggest challenge. To find a balance between what we live, feel and experience versus what we think. For this reason, the key to overcoming this disconnection is ***Heartfulness***, which means not only bringing the mind, but also the heart to the present moment, achieving a connection between both.

At the end of this chapter, we are going to share with you a very simple, but at the same time, very deep and effective exercise to achieve **coherence between your mind and your heart.** To keep these two energies and inner worlds (intuition and logic) in agreement, keeping them hand in hand, not controlling each other but going together in harmony.

But before we share this exercise with you, we want to give you a special gift: Seven Principles to transform your life. These seven principles are taken from the 14 fundamental principles of inner transformation of the *Huna Philosophy*, the mother of Ho'oponopono.

The **Huna philosophy** is an ancient way of life that connects our being with Nature and the universe in total agreement, without criticism or judgment, setting our attentive gaze on the present moment. This philosophy was born more than five thousand years ago in Polynesia and today, we take all its principles and universal laws using the **Ho'oponopono** technique. These seven principles will help you transform your life because they will help you **ground yourself** in the present moment and unleash your inner power.

First principle
Ike: The World Is What You Think It Is.

This principle (in Hawaiian: Ike) allows us to realize that the world is as we are, not as it really is. **The world is what we are**. If I believe that life is hard, difficult and complicated, that is what I will be manifesting into my life. If I feel that life is easy and that everything in life comes to me in a natural and fluid way, then that is what I will be experiencing. Life is whatever you think it is and it adapts to your belief system, to your values and thoughts.

Second principle
Kala: No Limits.

You have heard this before, but let's repeat it: You are an unlimited being. That means **there are no limits to what you wish to be or do in this life**. The only limits are set by you. You are the only person who draws the line and creates a ceiling on your desires and your dreams. But life has no limits. That means you can be and do whatever your heart guides you to be. So think about it for a moment. You are *limitless*. What would you like to do with your life today?

Third principle
Makia: Energy Flows Where Your Attention Goes.

Our attention is very powerful. We are going to give you a very practical example. Imagine you are standing in a dark room, completely surrounded in darkness. In your right hand, you hold a flashlight and turn it on so you can see what is in that room. The only problem is that you can only see what you focus your flashlight on. You cannot see everything in the room, but the only thing you will be able to see is what you are shining the light of your flashlight on. You will probably be able to see a wall and a corner of one of the rooms. But you will never know exactly how big the room is unless you turn around, unless you move. Love is the energy that gives you that power. Remember that fear leaves you stuck and rooted to the floor.

This is similar to how life manifests itself. We see what we focus on. But everything else is left in complete darkness, just like in the dark room. If we focus on thinking and believing that life is hard and difficult, that our economy is always damaged, that work is hard, that nobody values us, and that all the work we do is devalued, then that is what we will be seeing from the world. And that is what we are going to be manifesting in our lives constantly.

The only thing you have to do to change your life, to transform it, is to change the position of the flashlight. Focus it on another part of this dark room to be able to see a little bit further, to be able to see reality as it is, not as you think it is or as you fear it could be.

There is much more within us than what we are seeing. You are a limitless being. You have no limits. So why do you believe that your life is limited? Why do you think that your resources are limited? Why do you feel that your health is limited, that your body is limited, that you are flawed, that there are broken things inside of you? There is nothing broken inside of you. Those are incorrect thoughts that need to be corrected.

Fourth principle
Manawa: Now Is The Moment Of Power

This is one of our favorite principles. It does not matter what you have gone through or thought in the past. It does not matter if (yesterday or five minutes ago) you thought you were a failure, or that your finances were unsalvageable, or that your body was corrupt, or that maybe you were not connected with your spiritual world, or that maybe your family was very dysfunctional. That stops now because now is the moment of power. **There is no more powerful moment than here and now**. And this means that in this very moment, you have all the power to be able to transform your life. Do you want a harmonious, healthy family? You have it. Do you want a perfect body, perfect health? You got it. Do you want a healthy economy? You already have it. Starting today, you begin to use all your energy and focus on what you really want. Remember, you are an unlimited being and the moment of power is now.

Fifth principle
Aloha: To Love Is To Be Happy With

This principle, the Aloha principle, has to do with love and the expression of happiness with… The rest of the sentence is completed by you (you can go ahead and fill in the blank). You can be happy with someone. You can be happy with yourself, as in Mariana's story. You can be happy for being the person you are, for discovering what you are discovering at this moment in your life, for reconnecting with your health, for connecting with your spiritual world, with your deeper side. Whatever the reason, you can find yourself happy and love the happiness that is in you.

Sixth principle
Mana: All Power Comes From Within

This is another principle that we love. It is important that you understand that the light is within you. Let's go back to the example of the dark room. Who has the flashlight to illuminate the darkness? You do, in your right hand. All the power to transform your life comes *from you.*

We have talked about the power of the inner child. We have talked about self-discovery in the energies of your physical body. We have also mentioned the power of beliefs and thoughts. You see, everything is within you, and you have all the power to change whatever feels harmful in your life, causing discomfort to you or to the people you love. All you need is to realize that all this power belongs to you. It is yours. It is here. And it is now.

Seventh (and final) principle
Pono: Efficiency Is The Measure Of Truth

This means that in order to understand the truth, we must be *effective. We* must *take action.* If we want to live a truth that is abundant, then we must be abundant beings. There must be coherence within us. If we want a healthy life, then from today on, your focus has to be on healthy eating habits and healthy emotions. Because it is useless to have the desire, but not to act in order to turn that desire into reality. Remember, desire alone is useless because it becomes an expectation that many times is incongruent with our reality. It is not enough just to *wish* to be well. We must *act.* We must be effective in setting this desire into motion so that the universe manifests it perfectly at the perfect time. Do you want to truly live a complete transformation? Then start by treating yourself perfectly, by treating yourself with truth, with love, by being loving to yourself and to your body, and understanding that you already have all the power you need. You have the capacity to be happy, to transform your life, to have a healthy family, to enjoy your family instead of suffering from it, to enjoy your work instead of suffering from it, to enjoy your finances and enjoy what that brings to your life, to understand that you are a completely abundant person. But to begin with, you need *consistency.* Desire alone does not serve us well.

We want you to have these seven principles as your standard from today moving forward. The world is what you decide. You are an unlimited being. All your energy flows where you want it. Here and now. In your happiness, you find love. You already have all the power you longed for, it is within you and as you act on it, your desires will become a pure truth, a part of your reality.

Your intuition is the one that guides you beyond reason, thoughts, and expectations. **Your most intuitive part, your deepest part**, is the one that guides you in the right steps to take in life, the one that shows you that everything is fine, that you should not be afraid, that life is full of challenges, but that you have all the power to embrace and tackle them, to conquer your fear and to achieve everything you set out to attain. You came here to be happy, and you are unlimited. Make the most of it.

EXERCISE

We are now going to share with you the exercise of **cardiac coherence.** But first, we are going to tell you something that you may not know that is already a scientifically proven certainty: the brain and the heart are *linked* through the peripheral nervous system, and with this, we put an end to the eternal battle between heart and mind. Now that we know this reality, the only thing left to do is to make them work in a coordinated and harmonious way. How to achieve this? Very simple. We have learned this technique from a teacher and friend who is a specialist in Chinese medicine and neuroplasticity, and it is also a variation of one of the exercises recommended by the great **Dr. Gregg Braden** and designed by HeartMath, an organization dedicated to studying the power and intelligence of the heart.

Ready? Let's get coherent! :)

Step 1: Take at least 10 minutes of your time and choose a place or space where you can be in silence without being disturbed. Turn off all electronic devices nearby (yes, including your cell phone) and sit comfortably. Try to keep your back straight and spine aligned.

Step 2: Close your eyes and smile as big as you can. It is important not to drop the smile. Make an effort to keep smiling throughout the entire exercise. If you notice that your smile falls, bring it back up again.

Step 3: Breathe in and out gently through your nose deeply with as little effort as possible. Do this for a few seconds. Then, visualize the air going in and out **through your heart**. This part of the exercise can be confusing, but as you practice it, you will see how it comes more naturally. Practice makes perfect.

Step 4: Next, keeping your smile and feeling the air entering and leaving your heart, you will connect with the energy of Gratitude, feeling grateful for something you have or something that has happened to you or that you consider important in your life. If you prefer, you can connect directly with the pure energy of gratitude (without thinking of a particular person, thing or event).

Step 5: Keeping your smile and focusing on this feeling of gratitude, you will continue breathing for 5 more minutes. Then, you can open your eyes and connect with the present moment.

How do you feel now?

HEART COHERENCE EXERCISE

https://www.marianandpablo.com/heart-coherence-exercise

Chapter 8

"Forgiveness is for you because it frees you. It allows you to get out of the prison in which you find yourself."
- Louise Hay

Forgiveness is the end road of acceptance. It is a page-turning. Forgiveness means "lesson learned." It is the action and the result. It is a path, and it is the destination.

To forgive is to integrate all your parts and embrace them. To forgive is to let go because it no longer serves us. It is a goodbye that does not hurt. To forgive is to come home and take off our shoes to walk barefoot comfortably. Forgiveness is not a show of superiority to someone who is hurting us, but an act of love and transcendence.

Have you ever heard the phrase, *"I forgive, but I do not forget"*?

We have heard it many times throughout our lives, especially from our grandmothers. This, perhaps, is one of humanity's worst phrases. This phrase says that we always have to be expectant, looking over our shoulder, waiting for the next grievance, knowing that sooner or later, something bad is going to happen.

"I forgive, but I don't forget" is a phrase of our ego-based on fear and insecurity, on limiting beliefs. Another bad phrase is, *"Better the devil you know, than the good you do not know."* Do you find similarities between the two? **Failure to transcend a situation of pain anchors us in suffering.**

Remember the phrase, "*Pain is inevitable, but suffering is optional.*" Suffering is a *choice*. It condemns us to live in the past, dreading the moment of repeating a bad experience in the future. This phrase is attributed to Buddha. The enlightened master explained that life is like sailing on a raft, on a small stream, and from time to time touching one shore and then the other. One bank represents pain and the other pleasure. If we stay on the pain shore, we generate suffering, and if we stay on the pleasure shore, we generate addiction. Life, then, is a great adventure that must be lived to the fullest, without risking safe or already lived experiences, for fear of the uncertainty of what is to come and the unknown.

Many times we do not forgive a person because we want to be right. To prove that we were right, that our truth was the absolute truth and the only possible truth.

Let's try a very simple exercise. Right now, place your right hand over your heart and ask yourself, *In a situation of pain, conflict or a lot of stress, would you rather be right? Or would you rather be happy?*

You will never get the other person to think the same way you do. And that, instead of being frustrating, should be a reason to be grateful. It is a good thing that we all think differently! In diversity, there is knowledge, wisdom and true learning that leads us to reflection, understanding and, finally, evolution. **We are intertwined** and every conflict at work, with a partner or with your children, should make you happy because we all have different perceptions of life and through the experience of others, we come to understand the world more fully. We all manage to connect with love in different ways. Each of us connects with our inner child, with our values, our beliefs, our way of expressing love in a different and original way. Then, in diversity, there is enjoyment; the true happiness of being able to find meaningful learning in a loving way, understanding that each one of us came to learn something in particular.

I truly forgive you

There is an incredible phrase that has accompanied us for years and has always served us in times of crisis and conflict, especially regarding family arguments. It belongs to the great writer Louise Hay, "*I forgive you for not being what I wanted you to be. I forgive you and set you free and set myself free as well.*"

To be honest, we believe that the last phrase was a personal addition. But that does not matter. What does matter is the depth of the forgiveness concept that is achieved in this short and powerful sentence. According to Louise Hay, **forgiveness is an act of freedom**. It allows us to let go of what we are holding on to in our hearts and that hurts us.

Another very interesting concept is the relationship between forgiveness and expectations. When we say, "I forgive you for not being what I wanted you to be," we realize that we often get angry with people or offended by their behavior because it was not what we imagined or wished they would do.

When we use this phrase, we bring to our consciousness the fact that we are not responsible for -and cannot possibly control- the behaviors of others. We forgive that part of us that wished to have that control. We forgive that unrealistic image of the other person that we had created in our mind, with the ideal response we wanted to hear. And in doing so, we let go of the mental fantasies with forgiveness, **freeing both the other person and us**.

Let's talk a little more about forgiveness with a true story that connects with Ho'oponopono. The Ho'oponopono which has become known and popular today, is actually a special version created by one of the last masters in Huna philosophy **Morrnah Nalamaku Simeona**. This **Kahuna** (a title given in Hawaii to a priest, teacher or counselor) is used to attend to people's conflicts, to guide them in a healing process. But after a while, she decided to create the method of self-identity through Ho'oponopono.

This method proposes that each one of us is the master of our life and we do not need any guide, shaman or teacher to achieve inner healing, but only the knowledge of the technique to begin the process of healing our inner child and connecting with our higher self to erase the limiting memories that create moments of unhappiness in our life.

The famous Dr. Ihaleakala Hew Len meets Morrnah at one of his seminars. Maybe you have already heard this story, but it is really amazing. If so, we propose you reconnect with it to live it from a new place inside you. If this is the first time you are going to listen to it, then be prepared to be amazed.

Dr. Hew Len was not a great believer in the technique proposed by Morrnah and has confessed that he had to attend her seminars many, many times in order to grasp its true meaning. The amazing thing about this is Dr. Len's personal experience later on. He recounted that he had started working in a neuropsychiatric hospital that did not have a very good reputation. The patients used to be very violent, and the place employees never lasted very long due to the stress of working in such a place. Have you ever worked in a place that generated a lot of stress for you?

Dr. Len decided to implement a special practice during his working hours. He would lock himself in a hospital office for hours with the reports of all the patients in the hospital and observe them. Then, he would use a special prayer with each one. He did this during working hours every day. After a while, patients began to show improvement, reducing medication and even being discharged and leaving the neuropsychiatric facility for good. Even the employees, nurses and doctors commented that they were comfortable working there and kept their jobs. After a short time, the hospital had to close because all their patients had been discharged.

And here comes the million-dollar question, *What had Dr. Hew Len really done to heal the patients? How did they miraculously heal?* The answer he gave was very simple.

He said, "**I simply healed in myself what was generating these situations in the patients**. I would just sit in my office and observe each patient and heal what was inside of me that had resulted in this reality that the patient was experiencing."

Does it sound like magic or madness? The magic, actually, is that this was a true story. Ho'oponopono works on the beliefs we store from our childhood. The things we take as truths are actually thoughts and beliefs. And as Louise Hay says, any thought can be modified. The only problem is the size and weight we give to thoughts. That weight is what gives power to any thought that pops into our minds. *If my mom says it, it must be true,* we may have thought at one time or another. So even if mom says complete nonsense, if as children we heard it long enough, this thing we hear becomes a belief. And this belief is the lens through which we will look at the world, it is the flashlight with which we bring our world into light. We create our dark room and everything in it with our thoughts. That is why it is so important to be able to observe the thoughts we have.

95% of these thoughts are not even original, but are a repetition of thoughts that we had yesterday and the day before yesterday and the day before that, and that we have actually heard from a family member, or at work, or in the media.

It is essential to understand that judgment, criticism and blame lead to nothing. The only thing we can really do is to **free ourselves from the burden that these emotions generate by being more compassionate with ourselves.**

How many times have we judged ourselves for something we have said or done? And how many of those moments of guilt, humiliation or shame have we been able to let go of over the years? Very few, right? This happens because we tend not to forgive ourselves. It is easier to forgive on the outside than to forgive on the inside. And this is not true forgiveness.

Now, we are going to share with you a particular story of a student who has given us permission to share her story with you in this book.

> ### *Maria's Story*
>
> *Maria used to tell us what an amazing person her father was and how difficult her mother was. Her father was adored by everyone and her mother, few people could treat her. Her father always told her that she was the best at everything and that she could achieve anything she wanted. Her mother, on the other hand, kept telling her how bad she was and the mistakes she was constantly making. Nothing was good enough. Nothing was right. In addition, her mother was extremely strict to the point of resorting to physical violence and imparting fear.*
>
> *Maria said that when she became a mother, she decided to do with her children the opposite of what her mother had done with her as a child. The result of this decision was not ideal, as she was never able to set healthy limits for her children, allowing them to do whatever they wanted for fear of being hated by her children, perhaps in the same way that she once hated her mother.*

The interesting thing about this story, and what caught our attention the most, is that instead of emulating the footsteps of her father, whom she deeply admired, she preferred to be the opposite of what her mother had been with her.

Extremes are never healthy.

We must look at our experiences in their entirety in order to be aware of what we have experienced and what we choose to keep inside and then recycle it so as not to re-experience the event.

As we grow up, we tend to recreate the emotional environment of our childhood home, and we also tend to reproduce in our personal relationships the ones we experienced with our parents.

As we grow up, we tend to recreate the emotional environment of our childhood home.

EXERCISE

We are going to accompany you in a short reflection exercise in order to bring to light the essence of your parents that is inside you. It is important that you understand that what you feel about them is not really your parents, but your perception of them. Each of us, with our particular energy, perceives reality with different eyes and different hearts. It is important to see what is within us beyond the subjective truth. We seek to see how we have stored our experiences in our subconscious, what we have told our inner child.

Here we are not going to judge your parents, but to reveal *the image you have created* of them inside yourself. We will share with you a series of questions that we would like you to answer as honestly as possible. You can take as much time as you need, but it is important that you answer them.

You can also individualize the answers by expressing what each of your parents were like. If you have siblings, they can answer them individually and then compare the answers. They will surely be very surprised. Remember, we are not judging or criticizing here, but helping you to relieve a great burden.

All questions are in the past tense. You can answer them in the same way, thinking about your past or also in the present tense, describing your current situation with your parents.

1. What is the first memory that comes to mind when you think of your father?

2. What adjective would you use to describe your parents? (Remember that you can individualize. For example: Mom was caring and Dad was distant.)
3. Were your parents permissive or very strict?
4. What was their mood like?
5. Did you feel that you could count on them, tell them your problems?
6. Did you feel accompanied?
7. Did you used to feel safe and protected when you were with your parents?
8. When have you ever felt afraid of your parents?
9. Did you feel that your parents judged you or criticized you for what you did?
10. Did they support you in your decisions?
11. What was the relationship like? Did you feel they were close, distant, easy-going or impenetrable?
12. Did you admire your parents?
13. If you had to choose one emotion that your parents generated in you (anger, excitement, embarrassment, etc.), which one would it be?

After taking the time to answer these questions, we recommend the following:

Let's heal your inner self. Review the answers you have written and answer this last question. Do *you feel that any of these characteristics exist in you today? Is this the same way you treat your children or yourself?*

If you have answered honestly, you will most likely find common ground, common ground between your parents and the way you relate to each other. This is no accident. The way we have been raised has formed a subconscious programming that we have been repeating and repeating and repeating year after year. The best way to reprogram ourselves is to first become aware that this programming is within us.

Chapter 9

"The highest form of human intelligence is the ability to observe without judging."
- Jiddu Krishnamurti

Have you ever felt like throwing your career away and starting a new job? Have you ever thought about turning your life around and, for example, moving to another country and starting a new life in a new place with a new job? Have you ever thought that you are not in the right relationship? Or that your love relationship is going nowhere?

All of this is completely normal. It is important for you to know that. The mind, as we said, creates its expectations and when faced with life uncertainties, new things, conflicts or difficulties, it prefers to wipe the slate clean and recreate everything from scratch. Just as we think it is perfect for us.

But therein lies the secret. To understand that **uncertainty is part of the magic** and that, in reality, it is not necessary to move to a new country or change careers, but to connect with the present, understanding that we already have everything we need to be happy.

And here is a key that we are going to share with you and that is of utmost importance that you put into practice. It is a great power, and it is very effective. It is the power of **blessing.**

You may think that blessing is only present in the religious world or as a religious practice, but in reality, blessing *is much older* even than any religion. Blessing is a magical power that allows us to connect with all that we have to enjoy and opens the doors to all manifestations of creation.

A few years ago, at the end of a podcast we made, the person invited asked us why we had used the word "blessings" at the end of the recording. She was concerned, as she thought that listeners would be upset to interpret this word as something exclusively associated with religion. We explained that blessing something or someone has nothing to do with a religious practice, but with a deep connection to the moments experienced. Therefore, you too can use the blessing for what it truly is: a key to manifest whatever you desire.

Blessing is a magical power that allows us to connect with all that we have to enjoy and opens the doors to all manifestations of creation.

Etymologically, the word "bless"' comes from the Latin *benedicere* and means *"To invoke or ask for protection in favor of a person, a situation, a thing, etc."* This word is composed of *bene,* which means *"good,"* and *dicere,* "to say." To bless literally means "to say well," to say good, the opposite of cursing. When we curse, perhaps in a moment of anger, rage or frustration, we are doing just the same, but opposite and to our detriment. We are invoking low vibrational energies into our lives. What we attract is neither positive nor in favor of our well-being, but the contrary.

We want to share with you a technique that we have learned thanks to the Huna philosophy. This technique is extremely simple and incredibly powerful, but it does require a little effort on our part.

The Art Of Blessing

The art of blessing is an energy that has the power to transform your life and can help you manifest what you long for and desire. There are three important reasons why we should start using blessings in our lives.

1. When we focus our attention on a high vibration, that is, on **positive thoughts**, we are activating the creative force of the power of the universe.
2. We are able to focus our energy **inwards**.
3. Blessing others also works when we use the power of the blessing **outwardly,** blessing food, our family, our loved ones, etc.

We can expand this power to encompass all areas of our lives. Now that we have told you why it is so beneficial to use the art of blessing, we will now share the **four primary ways in which you can use it.**

Affirmation

If you wish to care for, increase and expand the life of someone or something, you can use an affirmation or statement. For example, *I bless the good health of my children. I bless my garden that nourishes me and my prosperity and abundance in life.*

Admiration

When you notice something that generates pleasure or well-being in your life, such as a sunrise or a beautiful evening, praising it or compliment it works as a kind of blessing. For example: What beautiful and blessed children I have! What a great day I have had today! What a blessed home I have!

Anticipation

When you focus on an event or situation that you have not yet experienced or has happened, you can use this type of blessing to anticipate its beneficial and positive outcome. For example, *What a beautiful family lunch we will have this weekend! I bless the work trip I will have next week. I bless the successful medical procedure I will have next month.*

<u>Appreciation</u>

When you feel grateful for something you have in your life, you can use this type of blessing to show your appreciation and gratitude. For example, you can use this type of blessing to show your appreciation and gratitude: *thank you for this beautiful moment shared with friends. I bless the food I will eat today. I bless the beautiful family I have.*

We highly recommend that from now on, you use this blessing tool every day to elevate your personal vibration with positive energy and gradually get rid of negativity. Remember, everything happens for a reason and everything can be a reason to be grateful because it has served as a learning experience.

Blessing opens the door to manifest in your life what you desire. But there is also another key thing you need to be able to turn your desires into reality and live the life you truly deserve—the second *Spiritual Law of Universal Success*. This second law that we want to share with you and that is incredibly powerful, The Law of Intention and Desire, explains that within every intention and every desire is **the power to manifest** them; that is, within every desire, there is also the power to make it come true.

As we mentioned earlier, desiring something and having the intention to achieve it is healthy. What we must avoid is having a rigid and immovable idea of how to achieve what we desire, since this process is part of the creative process of the universe. If you respect these laws, you will be able to have full confidence that what you desire will become a reality.

The blessing opens the door to manifest what you desire the most in life.

Have the intention and desire for something that you really want to live in your life: your strong body, your perfect health, your harmonious family, healthy relationships, your ideal job, etc. Everything you desire can be manifested. But remember, every desire must be released with the law of detachment, understanding that the universe will manifest it in the **perfect time and space.**

Perhaps this can be better understood with a story, so let's share with you the story of how Mariana met Pablo.

> ### Mariana's Story of a Wish Come True
>
> *Earlier I told you about the turning point in my life, the moment when I decided to start being happy.* **What I did not tell you is that the same day is when I met Pablo.** *That day, which had started with anguish and pain, gradually turned into the best day of my life. And I want to tell you why.*
>
> *I decided to go to the cooking course that my friend was teaching so I would have an excuse not to stay at home with my family. That day, walking,* **I decided to be happy.** *I understood that my parents only wanted the best for me, as did my brother, and that by wanting the best for me they had certain expectations of me. I also understood that this was not something harmful, that they were not really hurting me. As I was walking and realizing this truth, I also found another very important truth—I had to forgive them. But above all,* **I had to forgive myself** *because all these demands, more than from my parents, were my own. I was demanding of myself to be perfect. And what does it mean to be perfect? I was looking for a perfection that is unrealistic and even unreachable. We spend our lives trying to be perfect and we never achieve it, because we do not really realize that we already are. That we always were. That we were always perfect in everything we have ever been able to do.*

When I understood that my family only wanted my happiness, I understood that all I had to do in life was simply that: to be happy. From that day on, all the decisions I have made and continue to make every day are based on my happiness. That Sunday, as I walked to my cooking class, I began to cry. The tears were falling freely and steadily. I discovered that I had a lot of pain inside me, and I was finally getting it out of my heart and setting myself free. By the time I got to class, I felt light, content and calm. This truth had changed the foundation of my whole mind, but also of my heart.

In the workshop, I was the only young woman. I felt at ease among the other older women participating in the event. I felt that I was in a warm space of acceptance, enjoyment and tasting. Who doesn't like food? Who doesn't like to eat? I, coming from an Italian family, love food. For me, eating has always been a moment of joy, of connection with the taste of life. So far, everything was magical... until Pablo arrived.

When I saw him walk in, I realized that he was the person who was meant to be with me. I do not have many words to explain it and I hope to be as clear as possible to be able to share with you this experience that comes from the deepest part of my heart. When I heard Pablo's voice and looked into his eyes for the first time, I knew he was part of my destiny. And my first thought was, "Oh God! Not now! I don't want to, I don't want to, I don't want to!" This moment was for me. This was supposed to be the first day of my life because I had set my mind to it, and I did not want anyone but myself. However, as I watched Paul, something inside me settled and began to beat. Something came to life and breathed new life into me as well. There was a voice in my mind telling me, "He is the right person for you." And yet, even though it was the good wolf talking to me, I didn't want to hear it. The evil wolf was also whispering to me, "This person is going to end up hurting you for sure. It's sure to be another failed relationship that will leave you with your heart shattered into little pieces and you won't be able to glue it back together again." It was hard. I'm not going to lie to you, dear reader. It took me a long time to understand that Pablo had been sent my way by some unknown force in the universe. A kind and loving force. But I am glad that, in the end, I was able to push my fear aside to listen to my good wolf.

Pablo is now one of the most important people in my life. He is the father of my son and has been my partner and colleague for more than 12 years. It is beautiful to understand that sometimes we are destined to share our lives with people who help us grow and evolve. People who allow us to expand our consciousness and even bring out the best in us. We bring out the best in ourselves when we are in the right space at the right time. He was the answer to my prayer to be happy.

Today I still ask for the same thing every night before going to sleep. I ask to be happy every day that the universe guides me towards happiness and joy. And I also ask for guidance to also give love and help all the people who come into my life.

The fact that Pablo is still in my life today is not a coincidence. There are no coincidences in the universe, just casualties. Pablo is the answer to my wish. That is why I share this story with you because I had an intention and a desire that I threw into the universe with all my heart and with total detachment. That day I created my own mantra, "From today, I am happy. My life begins today. I am happy now." And that same day, only half an hour later, my and Pablo's paths crossed.

Four Healing Words

"We are here only to bring peace to our own life, and if we bring peace into our own life, everything around us finds its own place, its own rhythm and peace."
- **Morrnah Simeona Nalamaku**

In this chapter we have talked about the power of blessing and the importance of being able to connect with the force of blessing because it allows us to open doors, erase memories and focus our attention on all the good we have in this life. Remembering that the power is within us and that this is the moment to transform our lives.

We are also going to share with you an incredibly powerful technique called "The Four Healing Words." This is one of the techniques from the Ho'oponopono method to transform our lives. These four words are phrases, and they are: **I'm sorry - Please, forgive me - Thank you - I love you**. They have an immense power because they allow us to connect with forgiveness, with gratitude and with love. They are not spoken outwardly. We do not say them to the universe, nor do we say them to a particular person, but we say these four words to ourselves. These words are dedicated to those parts of us that may be in darkness, that may still be hurt or wounded, or that simply need more love. Being able to connect with love and forgiveness allows us to clean that place inside of us and understand that we are here to learn how to heal.

Every event in life is a learning experience and an adventure, and it has arrived for us to learn from it. **Most knowledge comes from mistakes and mistakes are not negative**; they are not failures, they are not God's faults. They are small achievements that we acquire in order to reach a new understanding in life.

It was not easy for Mariana to understand that her happiness was what mattered most. She felt that she had failed in all areas of her life: her family, studies, career, and work. But when she understood that happiness was in her hands, she realized that she had the power to grasp it. And, little by little, she noticed that all areas of her life were starting to heal.

Forgiveness is a key part of healing. It is important to forgive ourselves: to forgive anger, anguish and frustration, because it is all part of the healing process. Then it is important to connect with gratitude. Gratitude is one of the highest vibrational energies in the universe. Gratitude, love, acceptance, joy and bliss are the main ingredients with which all creation manifests and with which energy flows in an abundant and natural way. Fear, resentment, anger and anger block this energetic flow and bring into our lives low vibrational energies, creating more anguish, more fear, more anger and more resentment.

These four words that we give you today, from Ho'oponopono, can be repeated in the order you want, as many times as you want.

Gratitude, love, acceptance, joy and bliss are the main ingredients with which all creation is manifested.

You can take any situation in life and be grateful for what you have learned and experienced. You can use these four words in the following way:

I'm sorry, please, forgive me, thank you, I love you. I'm sorry, forgive me, thank you, I love you. I'm sorry for not recognizing how important (the situation) is to me. I appreciate this new opportunity to become aware of (something you consider you've learned) and the opportunity to share it with others. I'm grateful for all the people who were part of this new learning experience. Thank you. I love you.

Embark on a journey of healing and Unleash your inner strength to achieve balance in life with our Ho'oponopono Program. Join us now!

https://www.marianandpablo.com/hooponopono-program

Pablo's Story

A few pages ago, you read Mariana's story, now I am going to tell you my story. Shortly before I met her, I was feeling ecstatic for many reasons. One of which was that I am an opera singer, and I was about to premiere my first leading role as Papageno in Mozart's opera "The Magic Flute." I really felt a kind of bliss because I was doing what I wanted to do and what I love.

At that time, I did not live in a very commercial area, and I had heard that very close to my house, there was a small Ayurveda center. I could not believe it! I heard about an Ayurveda cooking class on a Sunday morning at ten o'clock and I thought, "I'm definitely going!" That Sunday, just a few days before the premiere of The Magic Flute, I arrived a few minutes late. As soon as I walked in, I saw sitting at the table, next to many older ladies, a very, very pretty woman and something made me feel that this girl was very special. During the class, I shamelessly flirted with this girl whose name was Mariana. With the class almost over, I confessed to one of the classmates that I was eager to get her phone number. A lady went out of her way to help me, and I finally got her email just before I left—she would not give me her phone number!

When Mariana was saying goodbye, I offered to take her home. At first she did not want to, and it was a little difficult to convince her, but I succeeded in the end. Well, actually, my classmates and I did. I immediately invited her to a world food fair nearby. We had an amazing time.

A funny thing I want to share with you is that, towards the end of the outing, I had ordered a delicious fruit smoothie and Mariana had ordered a horrendous one. After taking a few sips and enjoying my drink, I offered to exchange juices so she could try mine. Mariana never gave me back the smoothie and I had to keep her disgusting fruit smoothie while she savored mine, which was exquisite. It was worth it to meet such a wonderful woman.

> *Then, when we started our way back, we spent more than half an hour looking for the car because I, distracted by her sweetness, could not remember where I had left it. From that day on, I knew that Mariana was "the one." I knew I had a good chance of sharing the rest of my life with her. Thanks to God, thanks to the universe, thanks to coincidences, thanks to synchronicity and destiny, today we are still together, and our love is growing day by day.*

Connecting with Your Deepest Self

There is an easy way to connect with our deepest self, with our intuition, with who we really are—meditation. To meditate is to leave our minds blank. To meditate is to put the mind in black. To meditate is to focus. Meditation is the opposite of concentration. Meditation is not a simple process; it is only for those who follow a spiritual path. All these statements that you may have heard sometimes, are statements that try to unravel something that is impossible to understand from the point of view of the mind.

The meditation process is just that, a process. It is not an end or a destination, but it is a journey. Meditation is a practice that anyone can do at any age or time in life. And there are as many meditation techniques as there are human beings in the world. Maybe not as many, but there are many techniques, and they all point to the same thing: **To find inner happiness, to find ourselves, and to find that peaceful place within us.**

Meditation is neither an end nor a destination, but a journey.

Learning to meditate—and doing it regularly—allows us to find acceptance of ourselves and, therefore, of others. It is the best tool to stop thoughts that are often more harmful than positive, harmonize emotions, sleep better, relax, eat better, help good digestion, and have more energy, greater creativity, intuition and productivity in our work. Sounds good, right?

Whether you meditate or have never meditated, today we want to give you two small gifts. At the end of this chapter, we are going to share **guided meditations** that you can do in the comfort of your home at any time of the day.

It is best to practice a meditation technique twice a day for approximately 15 to 20 minutes before doing things and after having done them. That is, you can meditate in the morning before starting the day's work and then again in the evening once you've finished the day's activities.

The dirty rag

Let's try to explain what meditation is with the following analogy. Imagine that on one hand you have a very dirty cloth and under your feet, there is a stream of clear, clean water flowing constantly. Slowly, you dip the cloth into the stream and then pull it back up. Then you dip it back in and pull it out again. If you look at the rag, you will notice that it is still dirty, but not as dirty as before. Possibly the water from the stream has helped to remove some of the dirt.

In this metaphor, the dirty rag represents our mind covered with worries, anxieties, negative thoughts, fears, etc. The stream illustrates the process of meditation. Each time we dip the rag into the stream (each time we meditate), our mind begins to slowly release everything that was disturbing it— *limitations, fears, negative beliefs.*

Buddha was once asked, "What have you gained from meditation?"

He replied, "Nothing. However, I have lost anger, anxiety, depression, insecurity and fear of old age and death." With this sentence, we sum up a little of the essence of meditation.

To meditate is to find the way back home to our center, to our heart. A place where all is well and where there are no fears, no dangers, nothing to worry about.

Meditating is a gift, a token of love towards us to give us exactly what we need. And every meditation practice is different because every day, we are different people as we live new experiences.

> *"No man can cross the same river twice, because neither the man nor the water will be the same."*
> **- Heraclitus**

There are people who do not like to meditate because they find it difficult or simply because it bores them. When we hear these words, there is something inside us that saddens us because meditating is like looking in the mirror. It allows us to see what is happening inside us to better heal and bring calm and harmony to our self. And since we are different people every day, every meditation will be different. Do not expect to always have the same experiences because uncertainty is one of the keys to happiness.

If you are still not convinced about meditation, we are going to "sell" it to you by talking about its *physical* benefits:

- Relieves pain.
- Rejuvenates the body - both internally and externally.
- Strengthens the immune system.
- Helps reduce blood pressure.
- Reduces the risk of cardiovascular disease.
- Increases energy significantly.

Also, several studies have proven the direct benefit of daily meditation practice on a mental and *emotional* level:

- Stimulates creative thinking.
- Improves memory.

- Aids focused thinking.
- Promotes concentration.
- Helps develop emotional intelligence.
- Reduces stress.
- Helps overcome insomnia.
- Promotes positivity.
- Helps improve our relationships by being less reactive.
- Promotes healthy self-esteem

And on a *spiritual* level:

- Increases self-awareness.
- Helps develop compassion.
- Connects us to the present moment.
- Establishes a deep connection with life.
- Brings us happiness, peace, inner harmony.
- Helps us connect with our truest self, called soul, essence, Atman.

It is striking that "doing nothing" actually does so many things. That something invisible provides us with so many concrete benefits.

Now we are going to share with you a practical exercise for you to learn how to do a very, very simple meditation. The *So-Hum* meditation.

SO-HUM Meditation

So-Hum is the sound and manifestation of the breath. "*So*" connects us with the air that enters our body. It is the connection with divinity, with inspiration. To breathe in is to connect with the Creative Source of the Universe and with the vital energy of the Universe that keeps everything alive and allows healing. "*Hum*" refers to the air that comes out, an expiration, a release of air. To expire is a synonym for dying. And in this case, it refers to letting go of what you no longer need. We must let go of what does not serve the body (stress, anger, limiting thoughts and beliefs) so that it can be filled with life energy, inspirational energy, divine energy, and so on.

So-Hum also translates simply as "*I am.*" But its meaning is connected to our true nature, the one that connects with divinity in a breath of air beyond our body, our personality, career, job, etc. What do you want to be inspired by today? Just breathe.

EXERCISE 1

We are going to teach you in a simple and practical way how to perform the So-Hum meditation. As we shared with you earlier, this meditation is known worldwide and many people explain the mantra as *I am,* but in reality, its meaning is much deeper and although it has to do with our identity, it actually has more to do with an expansion of your consciousness and a connection with your true self.

When "*So*" enters the body, it enters with the energy of life and "*Hum*" lets the ego, our limited individuality, exit the body. This is the meaning of So-Hum.

When you inhale "*So*," you are inhaling life. When you breathe out "*Hum*," you are breathing out ego and limitation. And this meditation, when practiced correctly, leads to **the union of the individual with the universal cosmic consciousness**. You will go beyond thought, beyond time and space, beyond cause and effect. Your consciousness will empty and, in that emptiness, it will expand, and peace and joy will descend as a blessing upon your whole being.

Let's get to work

All you have to do is find a quiet place, in silence, to sit comfortably with your arms and legs uncrossed. Try to have at least 15 to 20 minutes without interruptions. Once you are comfortably seated, close your eyes. Begin to bring your attention to your breathing. Visualize how the air flows in and out effortlessly. Let your breathing flow smoothly, at your own pace.

Once you feel relaxed, the next step is to observe your thoughts without judging them. What does it mean to observe your thoughts? Just let them pass by without getting carried away with them. This process is similar to looking up at the sky to watch the clouds pass by. Simply watch your thoughts and observe how they come and go.

Then, you are going to introduce the mantra So-Hum. How? Very simple. When you inhale, you are going to think mentally, without effort and without sound, the word "*So.*" And when you exhale, the word "*Hum.*" Mentally and at your own pace, you will repeat "*So*" when you inhale and "*Hum*" when you exhale.

This process will take 10, 15 or 20 minutes—whatever you can manage today. If thoughts, body sensations or any other type of interference appear, all you have to do is return your attention to the mantra.

It may be difficult at first, but the important thing is to connect with the present moment with the help of the mantra and allow the thoughts to follow. Do not try to direct, block or deny them; simply observe them. Whenever you feel your attention wandering, just bring your attention back to the *So-Hum* mantra.

It is not advisable to use a timer or clock that wakes you up violently when the time is up. You can use the sound of a soft bell to indicate that the desired time has arrived. Once you finish, try to remain silent for a few minutes and then gently and softly open your eyes.

As time goes by, you will see how you can extend the time of this meditation. In the meantime, the ideal is to practice it twice a day or at least once a day.

SO HUM MEDITATION:

https://www.marianandpablo.com/so-hum-meditation

The Real "Why"

The purpose of meditation is to connect with who we really are and to stop identifying so much with our thoughts. To meditate is to let the cloud of toxic and negative thoughts dissipate and to glimpse at our inner spirit. At first, as we said, it may be difficult to control the maelstrom of thoughts. If you have never meditated, you may feel frustrated or anxious. But understand that this is just a thought and is part of the process. The goal of meditation is to connect with the space of the mind that is calm, to let go of thoughts in total tranquility and detachment.

The secret of meditation

Another key concept of meditation is that it makes us aware of a great secret of the universe—**we attract the reality we live.** There is no one to blame. There is only one person responsible for the life you have—you!

According to the **Law of Attraction**, you create your own reality by attracting into your life the same vibration that permeates your thoughts and beliefs. That is why it is so important that you bring attention to your belief system. And it is also crucial that you forgive yourself for attracting perhaps painful things into your life from a place of unconsciousness.

Now that you know these principles, you will pay more attention to what you think and what you wish for because sooner or later, it will come true. Be grateful; eliminate the poisons from your life; stop feeding the evil wolf; reprogram your mind with positive thoughts and breathe because now comes the most beautiful part.

Look at your life with new eyes

Visualize life as you really want to live it. It is time to imagine a blank canvas and start painting your life with the colors you choose. Today you will paint your life with exactly what you want, with what you feel you deserve, and we know, even without knowing you, that you deserve the best.

In the words of the poet Rumi, *"You are already everything you ever wanted to be."* You are the creator of your life, and you have everything you need to live an excellent, fulfilling and healthy life. You just need to learn how to focus your energy to bring it to you.

Exercise 2

After practicing the *So-Hum* meditation, you will now create a **Sankalpa**. Sankalpa is a Sanskrit word meaning *intention, purpose and determination*. A Sankalpa **is a personal mantra** that we create.

This is a vow, a promise that we assume with seriousness and commitment to ourselves. It is a short and positive phrase that works as a receptacle of the energy emanated in the practice of meditation to be used with an intention and a deep desire to improve any aspect of your life, to change a habit or even to heal personal relationships.

The purpose and objective of Sankalpa is **to transform our life patterns in a positive way**. The idea is to repeat a phrase that you like at least three times while you are in a meditative state. For this reason, it is important that you first perform the so hum meditation to connect with your deepest part, your true essence.

Once you finish the meditation, you will create your Sankalpa. Remember, it has to be a personal mantra that you create and that summarizes in very few words what you want to live in your life. Use positive words and verbs always in the present tense, not in the past or future tense. For example, *"I have a perfect job. My relationship with my partner is perfect. It is harmonious and surrounded by love. My body is perfect. It is the temple of my soul and is in perfect health."*

Whatever phrase you create, remember to repeat it three times after meditation and you cannot create a new one until it has manifested in your life. Imagine that this phrase is attracting to you all the creative force of the universe to manifest in your life. You can even use the words *here, now, in this moment, now in my life.*

Remember that the moment of power is now, it will not be tomorrow, and it was not yesterday. You have all the power now to transform your life. You have everything you need to be happy. So put together your most powerful phrase, your own sankalpa, the one that will attract all the creative energy of the Universe to manifest here, now in your life. If you wish, you can also write this personal mantra on a piece of paper and take it with you to your work or wherever you go. You can also have it somewhere in the house. A very interesting idea is to stick the personal mantra on a mirror. This way, every time you look into your eyes, you can repeat your power phrase, vibrating what you desire with all your heart.

Today you start a new life. From today you start to be happy.

Conclusion

The last key to healing your life is to integrate all that we have shared so far, and to do so, **love** must be present. Remember: no one is born knowing. No one knows what love really is. Each and every one of us has a different perception of the world, of reality and of love. That is why Louise Hay's phrase, as well as the four words that heal, are so powerful; because they allow us to understand that everything can be learned and that each one of us has things to work on and to heal. If you want to heal a relationship, you must have love. First, self-love and then feel love for the other person with whom you want to heal the conflict.

Many times we do not forgive for fear of being hurt again. Fear is the opposite of love, not hate. When we experience fear, we stay anchored to a past space. Fear paralyzes us and leaves us in a space of no change, no growth and no evolution.

If you are reading this book, it is because you want the opposite in your life—evolution, growth and change to live new and better experiences.

When you experience love, a love without conditions, without limits or judgments, without requirements, without prescriptions, then you live a magical, healthy and purely blissful life.

> *"What will survive of us is love."*
> **- Philip Larkin**

This phrase summarizes everything we have been sharing in this book. Love is the basis of all transformation. Self-love is what will open the door to your greatest transformation in life. It is the first step to your new life.

A wise doctor once said, "Every disease can be cured with love."

A skeptic rebuked him, "What if it does not work?"

The doctor replied, "Just increase the dosage." :)

In the middle of writing these pages, there were two events that transformed our lives forever and we want to share them with you at this moment to honor these people and also to celebrate this book that was a dream fulfilled for us.

Sergio Medina, to whom we have dedicated this book, left for a new life. We feel the need to tell you a little about him since he is the one who receives the dedication and also the one without whose presence and drive these pages would not have been written.

Sergito was a huge man in a small package. At 5'5", shorter than Mariana, he seemed to go unnoticed. Regardless of his height or physical build, he was one of those people who commanded the attention of an entire room. He was born on March 22, 1962. His mother, Mimi, told him that his father had died before he was born and for that reason, they were alone. But after his 13th birthday, he discovered a sad truth—his father was not dead. His mother did not want him in their lives for selfish reasons that we will not share here. The important thing is that Sergio was able to connect with his father, who had been looking for him for many, many years.

In short, his life was not perfect, nor was it very happy, but when he reached his 40s, he was able to turn all his anguish and sadness around and rebuild his life.

Sergito was an insurance promoter, a cab driver, worked in a radio station and created his own online radio station when it was not yet fashionable. He was a masseur, reflexologist, distributor of health products, Reiki master and so many other things. But what stands out the most is that Sergito was a GREAT PERSON, with capital letters. Sergito was a small person with a huge presence. He was also the person who united us in this path of learning and teaching.

He was our Reiki master at the Traditional Usui System school, and he was the one who taught us to connect with our inner power, **which is all-knowing, all-healing and all-balancing.**

Conversations with him were never boring and could last for hours, and between words, we found similar experiences in spite of our differences. Most of the conflicts we used to have in our lives were the same ones Sergio was going through in his, and thanks to his words and his way of seeing the world, we managed to harmonize ours. We like to think that we have done the same for him.

Sergito was the one who said, "Well, guys, now get ready, it is your turn to give workshops and courses." And despite our doubts and insecurities, we did it and it went great. Every workshop, every seminar and every course we have given was thanks to his drive and his decree.

We were and still are good teachers, not only because we have dedicated many years of study and improvement, but also because we have had the best teachers. He participated in almost all of our events and used to share his opinion with us afterwards, during a hearty dinner.

Sergio Medina was, for us, a father, teacher, brother and friend, but above all he was Sergito. Words are not enough to say how much we miss him. He accompanied us in everything we were doing. He was present at Pablo's opera and singing presentations, in our courses and seminars, in our retreats and our practices with students. He even accompanied us to the clinic for our weekly pregnancy check-ups and was the first to greet us from the sidewalk when Mariana was admitted for delivery.

Luckily, there are no things left unsaid. We always told him how much we loved him. The hugs to say hello and goodbye were the kind of hugs that last for a while. The messages always had a joke or something funny and the coffees we shared were the sweetest.

Definitely, there were no things left unsaid, but there were things left to do. There is a big list of things we would have loved to share with him. We would love it if our son, Noah, could have met him long enough to chat with him or play a fun game. Anyway, we are grateful that he was able to meet him. He will forever be a grandfather to our baby boy.

This may be the story of an ending, but it is really the story of a beginning...

The second event that transformed our life was our pregnancy and the arrival of Noah into our lives. Noah Dino was born on September 28, 2021, and from then on, we embarked on a new adventure. The adventure of being full-time parents. Noah enjoys our company 24 hours a day, 7 days a week, 365 days a year. We will tell you later if Noah considers this a joy or a punishment.

As parents, we are super proud and happy to have all our time for him and to love what we do. Day by day, we work to make our relationship healthy and harmonious and to express everything we feel to each other, with respect and awareness. We also continue to work individually, within ourselves, taming our inner demons, and feeding the good wolf at all times.

We know and understand that everything starts with you, that all the power is within you and that everything we need to be happy we already have it.

Neither Pablo makes Mariana happy, nor Mariana makes Pablo happy.

Each one of us is individually happy. We know that happiness is a decision and a responsibility, it is our only duty in this life. We understand that all Noah needs to be well is for his parents to be happy. And for him to be happy, he needs a healthy structure, respectful and positive communication, and a warm home that nurtures inner love. That is what we work to achieve day by day.

It is not magic. It is not something miraculous. It is work, and it is a commitment to oneself.

That is the commitment that you have also made by reading this book. And it is the commitment that we hope you have made by doing all the exercises that we recommend in this book.

This is the real key to any transformation: **commitment, respect and patience with oneself, self-love**, the **hope** that one can always be better, and understanding that everything is a learning process. Everything takes **time**.

To get rid of our demons and stop feeding the big evil wolf is not something that can be achieved overnight, but it is something that can be done, and it does transform us.

That is the **promise** of this book and each and every chapter. To help you consciously find the love to accomplish everything you want in this life.

All the power is inside

The moment of power is now. You are a work of art in progress. You are a superhero with superpowers. Allow yourself to discover all of your special powers. Give yourself the respect you deserve so you can appreciate all your little parts with awe, love and reverence. Celebrate who you are today.

Remember that today is the first day of your life. These same words that Mariana said to herself in a moment of insight, we give to you today.

Today your life begins. From today forward, you are ready to be happy. Today begins your new life. Enjoy!

For more information and to learn more about how we can help you achieve your own personal body, mind and spirit transformation, book a free discovery call here:

https://www.marianandpablo.com/discovery-call

THANK YOU FOR READING OUR BOOK!

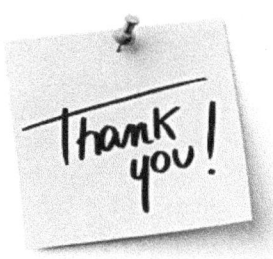

DOWNLOAD YOUR FREE GIFTS

Just to say thanks for buying and reading our book, we would like to give you a few free bonus gifts, no strings attached! Scan this QR Code or visit **https://www.MarianandPablo.com/PMFreegifts** to access your free gifts.

We appreciate your interest in our book, and we value your feedback as it helps us improve future versions of this book. We would appreciate it if you could leave your invaluable review on Amazon.com with your feedback. Thank you!

YOUR NEXT STEPS

BOOK A FREE DISCOVERY CALL WITH OUR TEAM TO LEARN MORE ABOUT GETTING YOUR OWN PERSONAL BODY, MIND AND SPIRIT TRANSFORMATION OVER THE NEXT 90 DAYS HERE:

https://www.marianandpablo.com/discovery-call

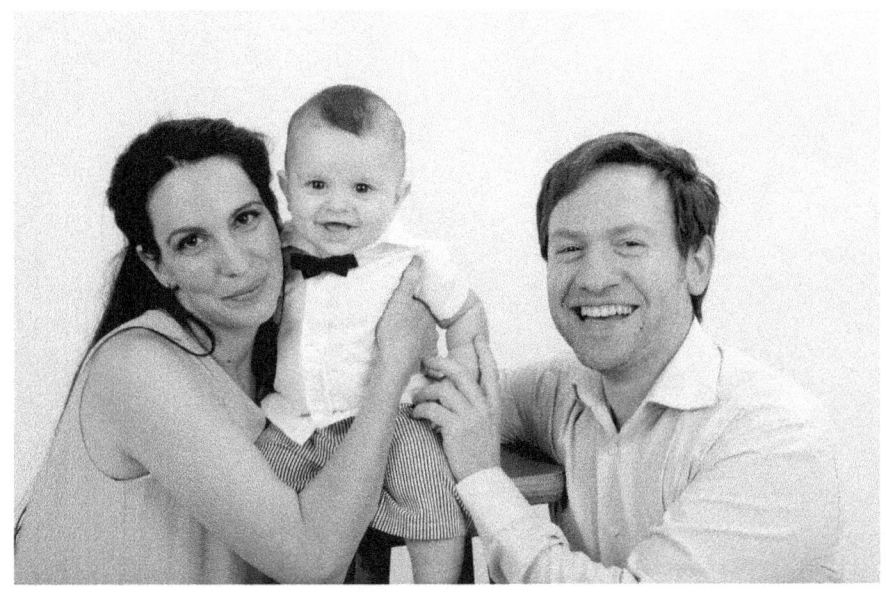

FREE RESOURCES

BREATHING EXERCISE

https://www.marianandpablo.com/square-breathing

https://www.marianandpablo.com/ayurvedic-test

https://www.marianandpablo.com/benefits-of-hot-water

https://www.marianandpablo.com/how-to-manage-pain-exercise

HEART COHERENCE EXERCISE

https://www.marianandpablo.com/heart-coherence-exercise

SO HUM MEDITATION:

https://www.marianandpablo.com/so-hum-meditation

HO'OPONOPONO PROGRAM

https://www.marianandpablo.com/hooponopono-program

AYURVEDA PROGRAM

https://www.marianandpablo.com/ayurveda-program

www.ingramcontent.com/pod-product-compliance
Lightning Source LLC
LaVergne TN
LVHW011422080426
835512LV00005B/205